Getting Research Published

An A to Z of publication strategy

Third Edition

Elizabeth Wager

Foreword by

Howard Bauchner, I<
Editor in Chief, *JAMA*
**and The *JAMA* Network

CRC Press
Taylor & Francis Group
Boca Raton London New York

CRC Press is an imprint of the
Taylor & Francis Group, an **informa** business

WITHDRAWN FROM
BRITISH MEDICAL ASSOCIATION
LI
0816683

CRC Press
Taylor & Francis Group
6000 Broken Sound Parkway NW, Suite 300
Boca Raton, FL 33487-2742

Printed on acid-free paper
Version Date: 20151123

International Standard Book Number-13: 978-1-78523-138-4 (Paperback)

Visit the Taylor & Francis Web site at
http://www.taylorandfrancis.com

and the CRC Press Web site at
http://www.crcpress.com

Contents

Foreword to third edition

In a rapidly changing world with soundbites, 140 character 'tweets', and over 7 billion mobile devices, the art and science of getting research papers published is more important than ever. Research that is poorly communicated is less likely to be published and, if published, more likely to be misunderstood. In this third edition of *Getting Research Published*, Elizabeth Wager updates her two previous editions.

This easy-to-read guide covers many topics, ranging from abstracts and blogs, to tables and trial registration. Many new important topics not covered in previous editions are included, such as predatory publishers, creative commons licenses, institutional repositories and journal cascades. Twenty years ago journals were delivered by mail, taking days to reach readers, now at a touch of a button articles are released to the world through social media, e-mail (electronic table of contents and other alerts), and often include video and audio. Knowing how to communicate in this technology-driven world of publishing is critically important.

Writing for journals and for other publications is more science than art. Although some authors are natural writers, for the vast majority it is a learned activity. Good writing is learned through reading, imitation, repetition, and instruction. The third edition of *Getting Research Published* successfully instructs in an authoritative, easy to use, and clear and concise manner. Take pen to paper, or in the 21st century more commonly fingertip to keyboard, with this book close at hand, and produce a well-written article.

Authors seek publication for numerous reasons, fame (promotion), fortune (grants), and simply to communicate their work. This A to Z of publication strategy should help all authors, young and old, novice and expert, in preparing manuscripts for journals and other publications, increasing the likelihood that their work will be published.

Howard Bauchner, MD
Editor in Chief, *JAMA* and The *JAMA* Network
October 2015

Foreword to second edition

Getting published is extremely important for a great many people. Promotion, grants, distinction, riches, and, as Freud put it in a more sexist age, 'fame and the love of beautiful women' can all flow from publication.

But there are also strong, less selfish reasons for publishing. We in rich countries overwhelmed with published material may forget that writing, publishing, critically reading, and debating are fundamental to any system that wants to improve – and certainly for any health system.

I'm writing this on a plane returning from Nigeria, and sadly Nigeria's health system might not unkindly be described as failed.

Joseph Ana, a friend of mine and the editor of *BMJ West Africa*, took over as health commissioner in Cross River State, one of the poorest states in Nigeria, 5 years ago, and after visiting every part of the region documented the dire state of the health system. It was failing at every level but especially at the primary care level where facilities were dilapidated and services barely functioning. People had no confidence in the system and went elsewhere to get care and give birth. Maternal mortality was 1%, childhood mortality 20%, and immunisation rates under 20%; and there were only 72 doctors for 3 million people.

Enhanced information flow will, Joseph believes, play an essential part in improving the health system. Indeed, a flow of good information and vigorous debate are in themselves an essential part of a well-functioning health system.

So there are very strong and unselfish reasons for publishing, but old lags like me, who have published and been rejected all over the place and roundly abused for some of the nonsense we've written, underestimate how terrifying and difficult it can be to get started in the publishing game.

This is where Liz Wager's book is so helpful. It provides a very readable and authoritative guide to every aspect of publishing in scientific journals, and the book's layout means that readers are both provided with a route map for publishing but can also find quickly information on the topics that might be bothering them. Perhaps the greatest tribute I can pay to the book is that I shamefully lifted some of the material for the workshop on publishing that I was running in Nigeria. The audience found the information extremely useful, and I thoroughly recommended the book to them – as I do to you.

Richard Smith
Former editor, *The BMJ*
Director, UnitedHealth Chronic Disease Initiative
January 2010

Foreword to first edition

Contemporary biomedical research has turned one traditional image of the scientist – the isolated figure, toiling alone, in a small, cluttered, dimly lit laboratory, late at night – into a quaint anachronism. The scale and complexity of today's research projects usually require large teams of people, who may be scattered across the world, with highly specialised skills. Despite the teamwork now inherent in most research, one part of the process, writing up the resulting paper, remains essentially a solitary undertaking.

This approach is curious indeed. Why venture into the wilds without a guide? Who thinks it's a good idea to light out for unknown territory without a map? Would you hand a scalpel to a novice and send him into the operating theatre alone? Of course not. This is, however, just the sort of experience plenty of junior researchers have once the trial is over, the experiments are done and the data have been analysed: they receive the earnest but empty directive to 'go write it up'. And here they may be following in the footsteps of their seniors, who probably navigated the publications process in a similar trial-and-error manner – doubtless heavier on the latter than on the former.

At last, help is at hand. *Getting Research Published: an A to Z of publication strategy* is a kind of guide for the perplexed. It will be useful to those who recognise they're perplexed by the process of writing and publishing, and helpful even to those who don't know what they don't know. (I even venture to suggest that we editors might learn a thing or two from it.) In this volume, Liz Wager provides just the sort of lively and intelligent guidance that will be warmly received by everyone who wants to publish research results. The format is user-friendly, the advice up to date, sound and tempered by pragmatism. Wager wears her considerable learning lightly, with a judicious selection of references and resources. Her recommendations are evidence based where possible, and qualified accordingly when evidence is lacking. As an active researcher, writer, teacher and advocate, she is highly qualified to synthesise and assess the literature of publishing research. Last, but hardly least, her enthusiasm and sense of humour are evident and most welcome.

Carrying out scientific research and seeing it into print are never going to be easy tasks. But by arming themselves with this guide, researchers can assure themselves of a better informed, easier and altogether more pleasant path to publication.

Faith McLellan
Former North American senior editor, *The Lancet*
President, Council of Science Editors
March 2005

About this book

This book has been written for everybody involved with getting biomedical and healthcare research published. Most of the book follows an A to Z format. I decided to arrange the information in this way because every publication poses different problems. I also hoped that this style would make the information relevant and accessible to readers with varying levels of experience and from different backgrounds, including individuals writing up their own research and people coordinating complex publication projects for research funders.

However, one problem with an A to Z format is that you need to have some idea of what to look for and it is not helpful for times when you don't know what you don't know. I have therefore included an overview at the beginning which contains a few longer sections to set the scene. If you are new to publications, I suggest you read the overview first and, if any terms are unfamiliar or any parts do not make sense, start diving into the rest of the book. Throughout the book, terms that appear in the A to Z are shown in **bold**.

I have not used references in the academic manner to support every statement but have included suggestions for further reading or useful websites within entries where this seemed helpful. Although some of the conventions of peer review date back to the 18th century, other aspects are evolving rapidly and, since starting to write the first edition in mid-2004 and updating it in 2009 and again in 2015, there have been several important developments affecting publications. I therefore urge readers to get into the habit of scanning major journals and keeping an eye on relevant websites (e.g. www.thepublicationplan.com) to stay up to date.

One reason for writing this book is that information about publishing research is scattered and some conventions seem never to have been written down. Many journal instructions to authors seem to hark back to a time when one or two collaborators wrote up their own small research projects and do not reflect the realities of large-scale multicentre trials. Another reason is that journals and meetings do not all function in a uniform way. With over 20 000 medical journals in existence, you would not be able to lift a volume that covered every requirement of every title, even if it had been possible to compile such a mammoth text. Many of the statements in this book are therefore generalisations. I have tried to guide readers around likely problems and offer solutions based on my experiences gathered over 20 years of writing, editing and coordinating publications for drug companies and individual researchers. I hope you find it helpful, but please remember to check the requirements of individual journals and meetings before assuming that I am right.

Elizabeth Wager
October 2015

About the author

Liz Wager is a freelance publications consultant, trainer, writer and editor. She has worked with doctors, drug companies, journal editors and writers on six continents. She is the co-editor-in-chief of *Research Integrity and Peer Review*, a fellow of the UK Enhancing the QUAlity and Transparency Of health Research (EQUATOR) Network Centre and visiting professor at the University of Split School of Medicine in Croatia. She studied zoology at Oxford and Reading but discovered she was better at writing about research than doing it. Before setting up her own company, Sideview, she worked for Blackwell Scientific Publications as an editor, was the medical writer for Janssen-Cilag in the UK, and then UK head of international medical publications at Glaxo Wellcome. Working in the pharmaceutical industry, she developed an interest in publication ethics and led a group that published 'Good Publication Practice for pharmaceutical companies' (*Current Medical Research & Opinion*, 2003). She chaired the Committee on Publication Ethics (COPE) from 2009 to 2012 and is a member of the ethics committees of the BMJ and the World Association of Medical Editors. She has done research into peer review (which, unlike zoology, does not involve operating temperamental equipment or washing-up) including Cochrane reviews on the effects of peer review and technical editing. She has written articles and book chapters on various aspects of scientific publishing and is a co-author of *How to Survive Peer Review* (BMJ Books, 2002). She lives in Buckinghamshire with her long-suffering husband and four tortoiseshell cats (who have to put up with her habit of reading medical journals in bed).

Sideview
Princes Risborough
E-mail: liz@sideview.demon.co.uk
Website: www.lizwager.com

Part one

Publication strategy – an overview

CHAPTER 1

Step-by-step guide to publication strategy

Most of this book does not follow a step-by-step approach because each publication will raise fresh issues and readers have different needs. If you already have questions or problems I suggest you use the A to Z section to find the information you need, but if you want a general overview the following steps are designed to help you navigate around the book and reflect the stages common to most research publications. **Bold** print indicates an entry in the A to Z section, which you should consult if you do not understand the term or want more detail.

1   *Identify the key message.* (What do you want the publication to say?) For example, your findings show that Tumorzap increases life expectancy in patients with advanced cancer. That is your **key message**. Remember that a message needs a verb (i.e. an action word, in this case 'increases'). A statement, without a verb, such as 'The efficacy of Tumorzap in advanced cancer', is not a message.

2   *Identify the **target audience(s)**.* (Who might be interested in your message?) The primary audience for this study would be oncologists, with a secondary audience of haematologists.

3   *Finalise the authors and **writing group** for this publication.* Ideally, you will have agreed some ground rules for **authorship** at the start of the study. The writing group may also include a professional writer who is usually not an author.

4   *Agree responsibilities for preparing and reviewing the publication.* Remember that more people than just the authors will probably need to review the publication before submission. For example, you may need sign-off from the research sponsor or approval from a head of department.

5   *Agree the **target journal** and a **second target** in case your paper is rejected by the first.* See **journal choice** for more details.

6   *Agree a timetable and a list of responsibilities.* (Who will do what?) Send these to all the **key people**.

7   *Prepare an **outline**.* This is especially helpful if several people are drafting different sections or if the paper is being prepared by a professional writer who is not an author. All authors should get a chance to comment on the outline and it is helpful to arrange a meeting or phone conference to allow discussion on this. Discussing the outline will save time and avoid disagreements later.

8   *Prepare the first draft.* There are plenty of books about **writing** but most start

from this stage. For successful, and pain-free, publishing, you also need to pay attention to steps 1 to 7.

9 *At the same time:*
- gather authors' comments, circulate them and prepare subsequent drafts. This process continues until you reach consensus. While you might feel exhilarated and excited when you prepare the first draft, you will almost certainly experience other times when you feel fed up, frustrated and demotivated. Resolving petty disagreements between **co-authors** or doing tedious jobs like organising references is never much fun, but keep your publication goal in mind. Although word processing and e-mail have revolutionised the process of circulating drafts, collating comments and redrafting papers, the disadvantage of electronic communication is that you may rarely speak to, let alone actually see, your co-authors. Picking up the telephone or having a face-to-face meeting may lift your spirits and renew your energy. It is also often the quickest way to resolve minor differences over wording and definitely preferable to endless e-mail 'ping-pong'. If at all possible, plan at least two **meetings** of the writing group: the first to discuss the data and agree the overall strategy (key message, target audience, etc.), the second to agree the final draft just before submission.
- consult (**internal review**). This goes on in parallel with the tasks in the previous bullet point. Who you need to consult depends on the nature of the research and how it was organised and funded. It also depends on the skills of the author(s) and writing group. Consider showing drafts to the following people.

Table 1.1: Internal reviewers

Reviewer	Focus of review
Statistician	Data presentation, statistics
Senior colleague	Methodology, presentation, journal preferences
Native English speaker	Language
Practising clinician not involved in research	Practical implications, discussion
Librarian/Information scientist	References
Naïve reader (partner, parent, friend)	Logical flow
Nitpicker	Annoying mistakes

10 *Prepare the submission package.* Draft the **covering letter** and make sure you have gathered everything you need for submission. This might include (depending on the journal):
- **copyright** transfer form
- signed declarations of **authorship**
- signed statements from everyone listed in the **acknowledgements** section

- statements on **competing interest**
- **permissions** to reproduce figures.

Check the title page for: author **names**, qualifications, **affiliations**, full contact details for **corresponding author**, details of individual contributions. Recheck the journal's instructions for other bits and pieces you might have forgotten such as: **key words**, **running title**, word count.

Check the journal's requirements for things like page numbering, justification (e.g. ragged right-hand text edge) and page breaks.

11 *Submit the paper.* But only after everybody is happy with it … and don't forget to let the key people know that the paper has been submitted.

12 *Wait patiently.* Or start work on your next publication.

13 *(unlucky for some …) The decision.* Inform everybody as soon as you get a decision. If it is a rejection, consider the reviewers' comments and revise the paper if they have identified remediable problems or simple mistakes, but do not waste time feeling dejected. Get agreement on any revisions and submit to the second **target journal** as soon as possible.

If you get a **conditional acceptance**, discuss the reviewers' comments with all authors and agree a response. Revise the manuscript and make a list of the changes you have made. Agree the revisions, then resubmit.

14 *Acceptance.* At last, all that work has paid off. You can now quote the paper as being 'in press'.

15 *Wait patiently (again).* How long you have to wait will depend a great deal on your **journal choice**. The period between acceptance and publication is known as the **lead time**. Use it constructively to agree how many **offprints** to order (*see* step 17).

16 *Check proofs*. These will be sent to the **corresponding author**.

17 *Order offprints.* An offprint form is often sent out with the proofs and will need to be returned without delay. To save time, find out how much offprints cost and agree how many everybody wants as soon as the paper has been accepted. Offprints ordered at the time of publication are usually cheaper than **reprints** ordered later.

18 *Publication.* Relish the moment! Your strategy has been successful. Bask in the glory and recommend this book to somebody else if it has been helpful!

19 *Follow-up.* Be prepared to respond to correspondence published in the journal. If readers (or you) spot a mistake contact the editor to discuss publishing a **correction (erratum)**. Send out **reprints** or electronic copies to people who request them.

20 *Evaluate.* Learn from your successes, failures and mistakes. Even a rejection or a tedious wait gives you information about what to do next time. If you are licking your wounds from a particularly unpleasant dispute about authorship or smarting from torrents of abuse from a disgruntled author (or editor), think about what you might have done differently to prevent these situations from arising. If you are handling a lot of publications, keep notes of **journal decision times** and **lead times**. These will build up into a useful resource for the next time you choose a target journal.

CHAPTER 2

Developing a publication plan for a multicentre study

Ideally, publication plans should be developed at the earliest stages of trial planning. Thinking about potential publications as you design the protocol can increase your chances of producing publishable results. Early planning and clear communication can also prevent later problems with authorship.

For large, multicentre studies, it is unfeasible for all investigators to be named as authors on publications. It is therefore helpful to agree **authorship** criteria at the start of the study. This will avoid many problems caused by unrealistic **expectations** or misunderstandings. At the outset, it may not be possible to predict exactly who will qualify as authors, but it is usually possible to agree how authorship will be allotted. The protocol development team (which usually comprises clinicians or senior scientists from the sponsor, a statistician and three or four key investigators) is a good starting point for a **writing group**, but, in the course of the study, personnel may change, so you cannot necessarily predict the exact composition of the final group, nor exactly who will qualify as authors.

Ground rules for invitation to join a writing team might be:

- protocol development team plus one investigator from each centre (to be nominated by each centre), or
- principal investigator, statistician, plus top recruiting investigator from each country, or
- principal investigator, five top recruiting investigators, plus company employees who meet International Committee of Medical Journal Editors (ICMJE) criteria.

Authors' responsibilities should be discussed and agreed at the outset. An invitation to join a writing team should not be viewed as an automatic qualification for authorship. Authors must expect to contribute to data interpretation and developing the publication.

Ground rules for authorship should be clearly communicated to everybody involved with the study, so that disagreements can be resolved promptly, and everybody has the same expectations.

Some companies and, to a lesser extent, academic institutions have their own authorship policies. These may be helpful (you should certainly be aware of them) but, if you consider the policy contravenes journal authorship criteria, such as the **International Committee of Medical Journal Editors (ICMJE)** criteria, you should be prepared to challenge them.

Authorship policies that may fall foul of accepted criteria include:

- never permitting employees to be named as authors on papers relating to company products
- only permitting a set number of employees to be named as authors (e.g. one per paper)
- always requiring an employee or particular individual (e.g. head of department, or professor) to be included as an author.

Such policies are likely to create problems of **ghost** or **guest authors**. It is much better to agree ground rules for each study.

Thinking about publications can also help with the study design. Imagining how the results might appear in a journal, or anticipating reviewer comments, may help to identify weaknesses and omissions. Involving patients or carers in clinical trial design is good practice, and may also help to identify interesting publications or increase the scope of potential publications, e.g. by including a quality of life assessment.

Publication strategies (and especially plans for authorship) should be clearly set out and communicated, preferably in writing, within the **investigators' agreement** or as a separate **publication agreement**.

Identifying target meetings can help to plan study timing – although this inevitably involves some crystal ball gazing, so you should not expect to be too precise. However, aiming to submit an abstract by a certain deadline may help to focus minds. If you wait to create your strategy until the data are ready, you might find you have needlessly missed a crucial deadline by a few days. Thinking about likely publications may also help to develop the **data analysis plan**, e.g. by identifying sub-group analyses at the outset.

An example of an outline publication strategy at the start of a study is shown in Table 2.1.

Once the results are available, the plan can be refined. At this stage, you should identify the authors, **key messages** and target meeting/journal for each publication. An example is given in Table 2.2.

You should also produce a detailed timetable and circulate it to everybody who will be involved with the publication. Agreeing a timetable is particularly crucial if you have tight deadlines to meet. A detailed timetable also increases your chance of meeting deadlines by setting out the steps to publication. These steps will vary depending on the complexity of the publication (which will affect how many drafts and review rounds you might need) and the study sponsor/organisers (who will have different requirements for review and approval).

If several people, or several organisations, are involved in developing a publication, a detailed plan can also be helpful in identifying who is responsible for each action or stage. A possible plan is shown in Table 2.3.

Table 2.1: Outline publication strategy prepared at the start of a study

Publication	Topic	Meeting/journal	Target audience	Submission deadline/ target	Publication date
Abstract 1	Efficacy data	ESMO	Oncologists	May 16	Nov. 16
Abstract 2	Safety data	ESMO	Oncologists	May 16	Nov. 16
Abstract 3	Sub-group data (haem)	EHA	Haematologists	Jan. 17	June 17
Abstract 4	Quality of life	*Cancer Nursing*	Oncology nurses	Feb. 17	Aug. 17
Main paper	Main results	Oncology (?*JCO*)	Oncologists	Q3 16	Q1 17
Paper 2	Sub-group analyses	Haematology (?*Blood*)	Haematologists	Q1 17	Q3 17
Paper 3	Long-term follow-up	Oncology	Oncologists	2018	?

(Q = quarter; thus Q3 16 indicates the third quarter of 2016)

Table 2.2: More detailed plan prepared when results are available

Publication	Key message	Authors	Meeting/ journal
Abstract 1	Tumorzap increases survival in cancer patients	X, Y, Z	ESMO
Abstract 2	Tumorzap causes less nausea than Chemowiz	Y, Z, X	ESMO
Abstract 3	Tumorzap induces complete remission in some haematological malignancies	Z, X, H	EHA
Abstract 4	Tumorzap improves patient quality of life	X, Y, Q	*Cancer Nursing*
Main paper (P1)	Tumorzap increases survival and is well tolerated in patients with advanced cancer	X, Y, H, Q, Z	*JCO*
Paper 2	Tumorzap induces complete remission in some haematological malignancies	Z, X, H	*Blood*
Paper 3	Long-term (two-year) follow-up confirms survival benefit with Tumorzap	Y, X, Z	*Ann. Onc.*

Table 2.3: Detailed publication plan showing timelines and responsibilities

Publication	Data ready	1st draft	Writing group review	Collate comments write 2nd draft	Xth draft …	Internal company review	All authors final review	Submit	Decision expected	Publication expected	Current status
A1	5 April (Stats)	15 April AW	30 April	5 May AW	…	10 May SM	12 May	15 May PA	July	30 Oct. 16	Submitted
P1	5 April (Stats)	5 May AW	26 May	10 June AW	…	1 July SM	10 July	17 July CA	Mid-Sept.	Jan. 17	Drafted

Key: AW = a writer; SM = senior medic; PA = presenting author; CA = **corresponding author**

CHAPTER 3

How long will it take?

Converting your publication strategy into a realistic plan requires some surprising skills. If you bought this book hoping that it would have handy tables showing exactly how long everything will take, you may be disappointed. It is possible to give broad estimates, but each publication is different and the timetable will depend on all sorts of intangible things like whether the authors work well together and how much priority the **key players** give to (and therefore how much time and resources they are prepared to invest in) the publication.

However, there are two tricks to publication planning. The first is to make the plan as detailed as possible. The second is to be as pessimistic as possible. (If you recall *Winnie the Pooh*: when planning your publication, try to be like Eeyore, who was sure that everything would go wrong, and save any bouncy, Tiggerish tendencies for later.) Breaking the plan into small chunks should ensure that you have not omitted any vital stages. It also means that you will quickly realise if timings slip and might be able to do something about it (or, at the very least, adjust the other timings). A recipe for disaster is a 'plan' (it hardly deserves the name) that simply states that the study data will be available in April 2018 and the primary paper will be published in September 2018. Given the right choice of journal and an extraordinarily dedicated and cooperative bunch of authors, this timing might be possible, but, to be of any use, a plan must break down the stages, otherwise you cannot tell anything is amiss until you miss your target publication date, and it is too late.

Chapter 2 'Developing a publication plan for a multicentre study' (pp. 7–11) should give you some ideas of the stages you need to include. The most obvious ones are:

- form a **writing group** and agree **key message(s)**, **target audience** and target meeting(s)/journal
- prepare an **outline**
- get agreement on the **outline** from all **key players**
- prepare first draft
- circulate draft and collate comments
- consult with people outside the writing group (**informal review**)
- continue process until consensus is reached (this stage is by far the most unpredictable and can drag on for ages)
- get approval to submit (this usually involves review by sponsor and/or institution)

- prepare submission package (**covering letter**, **permissions**, etc.)
- submit publication
- receive decision and reviewers' comments
- either respond to comments (if you get a **conditional acceptance**) or submit to second target journal if your paper is rejected
- receive acceptance
- check **proofs** and order **offprints**
- celebrate the publication!

Surprisingly, preparing the first draft is often relatively straightforward, especially if you are working from a well-prepared protocol and statistical report. However, here are some stages that could trip you up:

- obtaining permission for reproducing **figures** and tables from other publications
- getting figures professionally drawn
- gathering all the information needed for the submission package
- internal review by the sponsor.

Did I hear a faint howl of anguish, or at least a slight muttering when I wrote that this book would not contain handy tables? The point I am trying to make is that, to be realistic, each plan must take account of all the factors affecting each individual publication and that a 'one-size-fits-all' approach (e.g. 6 months to publish any paper) is doomed to failure: but here are a few tables.

Table 3.1: Timing for pre-submission stages for an 'average' research paper

Stage	Best case	Average	But it could take ...
Organise meeting, agree strategy	1 week	4 weeks	3 months
Prepare outline	1 week	2 weeks	1 month
Agree outline	1 week	2 weeks	1 month
Prepare first draft	2 weeks	4 weeks	3 months
Consult/reach consensus	4 weeks	10 weeks	4 months
Internal review/approval	2 weeks	4 weeks	3 months
Prepare submission package/submit	1 week	2 weeks	2 months
Total	**3 months**	**7 months**	**17 months**

Table 3.2: Timing for abstracts

Stage	Speedy	Sluggish
Agree strategy	1 week	4 weeks
Prepare first draft	1 week	2 weeks
Consult/reach consensus	2 weeks	4 weeks
Internal review/approval	2 weeks	4 weeks
Submit	1 day	1 week
Total	**6 weeks +**	**15 weeks**

Table 3.3: How long do journals take?

Stage	Rapid[1]	Fast track[2]	Moderate[3]	Dinosaur[4]
Decision – reject	2–10 days		1–3 months	3–6 months
Decision – accept	2–4 weeks	1–3 days	3–4 months	3–6 months
Allow time to respond to reviewers' comments – that's up to you!				
Final acceptance	1 week		1 month	3 months
Lead time (acceptance to publication) – web[5]	1–5 days		Variable	6–12 months
Lead time – printed version	4 weeks		3–4 months	6–12 months
Total (acceptance to publication)	3–12 weeks	4 weeks	7–9 months	12–21 months

1 Examples of rapid publications are journals such as *Current Medical Research & Opinion* or expedited review in the *International Journal of Clinical Practice*.

2 This applies to *The BMJ* and *The Lancet* **fast-track**.

3 Moderate – this mainly applies to weekly journals, such as *The BMJ* and *The Lancet* (regular, not fast-track).

4 Dinosaur – this applies to many specialty journals – the lower figures generally apply to monthly journals and the higher figures to less frequent (e.g. quarterly) journals, but there are exceptions.

5 Many journals publish on their website before the print version. The time to web publication is not included in the total figure, because it does not affect the lead time to printing. For purely electronic journals, e.g. *PLOS Medicine* and all the BioMed Central journals, there is no printed version, so final publication occurs on the web.

Research your target journal carefully to find out where it fits. The important message of this table is that **journal choice** is often the most important factor in determining the speed of publication.

■ How long do conferences take?

Abstracts are either rejected or accepted; there is no messing around with conditional acceptances or responding to reviewers' comments. The meeting dates are fixed, but there is considerable variation in submission deadlines.

Table 3.4: Timings for conferences

	Small/regional meeting or 'late breaker'[1]	Major international meeting
Time to decision	1–3 months	2–4 months
Time from acceptance to meeting	1–3 months	4–8 months
Total from submission deadline to meeting	2–6 months	4–12 months

1 Some large meetings permit **'late breaker' abstracts** – this is the equivalent of the journal fast-track and is usually reserved for new and interesting data.

■ General rules

Once you have worked on several publications with a core group, you will get a feel for how long they usually take. It is much harder to estimate how long a publication will take to develop if the writing group has not worked together before. A number of factors will influence the timetable and, while you cannot usually do anything to change these, at least you can take them into account if you are trying to plan, as shown in Table 3.5.

Table 3.5: Factors affecting the time it takes to develop a publication

Factors encouraging rapid publication	Factors that tend to slow down publication
Small writing group (< six people)	Large writing group (≥ six people)
Writing group members can meet easily	It is difficult/costly to arrange meetings (e.g. members are in different time zones)
Stable membership of group/other players	Writing group members have not worked together before, or do not get on well
Writing and publication experience	Lack of publication experience
Writing group members know and like each other	Changing personnel throughout study and while developing publication (e.g. statisticians, writers, sponsor representatives)

(continued)

Factors encouraging rapid publication	Factors that tend to slow down publication
Effective leadership of writing group (e.g. inspirational principal investigator)	Tension within writing group (e.g. battles for seniority or several people with strong and differing opinions)
Straightforward methods (e.g. similar design has been published before)	New design or complex study
Straightforward results (i.e. clear interpretation, everybody agrees on what they mean)	Controversial or inconclusive results/lack of agreement about interpretation
All key players give the publication high priority	Publication has low priority for some players or priority keeps changing

CHAPTER 4

Working with a medical writer

Professional medical writers are often involved in developing publications, especially those reporting industry-funded research. Some investigators and journal editors are uncomfortable about this practice, considering that it may encourage undue influence by the trial sponsor in presenting the results and introducing bias, or may lead to problems of **ghost** and **guest authorship**. However, others recognise professional writers as facilitators who can raise the standard of publications, ensure relevant guidelines are followed, and make the whole process simpler and quicker.

Having spent over 15 years earning my living as a medical writer, it will not be hard for readers to work out which view I believe is correct. However, in this chapter I will attempt to suppress my prejudices and consider the potential benefits and disadvantages of involving a professional writer.

■ Advantages of involving a medical writer

A good writer will bring the following skills and attributes to a project:

- excellent command of English
- expertise in preparing publications and presenting scientific data
- familiarity with journal requirements and preferences
- realistic ideas about chances of acceptance at different journals
- familiarity with guidelines such as **CONSORT**, **International Committee of Medical Journal Editors (ICMJE)** Recommendations, **Good Publication Practice (GPP3)** for publishing company-sponsored medical research
- experience of dealing with journals, e.g. responding to reviewers' comments
- coordination and project management skills
- expertise in preparing **figures** or professional contacts for getting this done
- access to tools that make writing easier, e.g. software for creating references
- uninterrupted time to write (unlike most busy clinicians, a writer can offer dedicated writing time rather than having to fit writing around other commitments – this alone can often accelerate a project)
- ability to take an objective view of data – it is sometimes easier for an outsider to assess results and, in particular, focus a publication by deciding what to

leave out, than for the researcher who has focused exclusively on the project for some time.

Being an outsider (i.e. someone who has not taken part in the research), the writer may also be more aware of differences of opinion within the group than the members themselves (who have grown accustomed to each other's idiosyncrasies). The process of briefing a writer may also provide a focus for discussing all the elements of the publication (e.g. **journal choice**, **key messages**) which might otherwise not be discussed (since junior members of the group might accept suggestions from more senior members without challenging them). A full-time writer may also have more experience than the team members in preparing publications and therefore be able to advise on strategy and how to avoid common pitfalls.

◼ Disadvantages of involving a medical writer

- *Money*: somebody has to pay the writer. This can cause problems if you have no budget for this or if the payment links the writer too strongly with the sponsor.
- *Lack of specialist knowledge*: most medical writers are generalists – they cannot be specialists in every field; however, they are experts in presenting data and preparing publications. This means that you should not expect the writer to be familiar with the complete literature around a subject. Some writers do specialise and develop considerable knowledge in certain areas, or may be familiar with the literature from having recently prepared a related article, but you should not assume this.
- *Acknowledgement*: in most cases when a writer works from a study report, or prepares an outline and then a draft only after discussion with the investigators, the writer will not meet the ICMJE criteria for authorship, since s/he will not have been involved in study design, data collection, analysis or interpretation. However, the last category is open to a range of interpretation, and, if writers get involved early in a study (e.g. in writing the protocol) or work from data tables rather than a report, they might qualify for authorship. This may raise questions about how the writer is acknowledged. If the **target journal** lists individuals' contributions to a study (rather than a traditional author list), omitting the writer from the list might raise queries from the editor, especially if this means that the person who prepared the first draft is not included in the list of contributors/authors. I personally feel it is quite acceptable for a medical writer to prepare a first draft of a paper and not to qualify as an author, since I prefer to apply the general rule that authors should be able to take public responsibility for the research (not just for the writing), rather than the criteria of exactly who did what. However, some journal editors may consider that this is **ghost authorship**.

■ Other points to consider

The job description 'medical writer' should not be interpreted too narrowly – some of the skills that a professional writer brings to a writing group are those of project management and coordination. A good writer will be able to guide discussions at writing group meetings, ensure that all the issues (e.g. target journal, **order of authors**) have been addressed and help the group achieve consensus. This coordinating role can be particularly helpful when authors are unable to meet because of distance or time constraints.

Paradoxically, authors and other writing group members will probably get the most from working with a professional writer if they remember the writer's limitations. Medical writers are usually good communicators with a broad biomedical background. They are not specialists and they are not telepathic. Time spent briefing the writer in the early stages is always a good investment. This process, in itself, may also be helpful, since it provides an opportunity for the group to discuss the important elements (such as key messages and target audience) together. Such discussion might not take place at all if the principal investigator prepares a draft and simply circulates it to all authors for comments (which is common practice in academic projects).

For this reason (whether a writer is involved or not), it is usually a good idea to circulate an outline before preparing a draft. When working with a professional writer, the authors need to provide especially detailed input to the introduction and discussion sections. If the key messages have been agreed, and a detailed protocol and data tables are available, the writer should be able to produce a competent first draft of the methods and results without much assistance, but it is unrealistic to expect a writer alone to develop the other sections which require a detailed knowledge of the existing literature and an understanding of the clinical implications of the findings.

Once a draft has been circulated, it is usually the writer's task to collate comments. The simplest method is often to use the 'Track Changes' function on your word processor. This not only highlights the changes but indicates who has made them. However, if changes are extensive, the resulting draft can get very messy and hard to read. Also, most software is not good at showing where sentences or paragraphs have simply been reordered, since there is no way of distinguishing a moved paragraph from one that has been rewritten. Specialised publication planning software may also be used to collate comments via a web-based system.

It may be possible for the writer to prepare a revised draft, incorporating all the comments, which is acceptable to all the authors. However, circulating drafts may reveal more fundamental differences in interpreting results, or varying views about how findings should best be presented. In this case, it is unreasonable to expect the writer to act as arbitrator. The best course is for the authors to settle their differences among themselves and then report the outcome to the writer. Similarly, it is unfair to expect writers to act as mediators in disagreements between sponsors and investigators.

CHAPTER 5

Dr Seymour and the disappearing paper: a cautionary tale

One stormy evening, three shadowy figures emerged from a brooding gothic tower overlooking a fetid swamp. Together they had hatched a plot to study Horrormycin, the latest product to emerge from the malodorous laboratories of the Darke Drug Corporation. These three schemers were Dr Procter, an ambitious medic, Mrs Countem, a buxom statistician, and Miss Plannem, a lowly study manager. Through mystical powers of telepathy and technology they had also consulted the sagely Professor Knowitall and the wealthy but indolent Dr Donothing. After days locked in the smoke-filled labyrinth, they blinked in the weak November twilight, their weariness overcome by the smug feeling that they had produced a masterly protocol for a study that would guarantee the success of Horrormycin.

After much grinding and refining in the forges of the legal and regulatory gnomes, the protocol was polished to perfection and the study began after receiving approval from the committee of fire-breathing ethics dragons. Three months later, Professor Knowitall was struck by the palsy and retired to his castle. In March, Dr Procter met an awfully nice chap on the golf course who told him about a job at Potions Inc. offering twice his current salary, so he left the Darke Corporation. And, being springtime, Mr Countem felt the sap rise in his veins, and soon Mrs Countem was on maternity leave.

As autumn approached and the leaves began to fall, the study ended. Miss Plannem, who had managed to keep the study within budget, was rewarded by promotion to a different department, based in a distant land. The data were analysed, in Mrs Countem's absence, by the inscrutable Dr Chi. Medical queries were handled in a desultory manner by the younger but even more ambitious Dr Climber, who was now responsible for Horrormycin but whose main passion was Bustergut, rapidly emerging as a panacea that might make the Darke Corporation rich beyond even the wildest dreams of its directors. The job of preparing the study report from Dr Chi's inscrutable, and somewhat incomprehensible, statistics was given to the shy and humble Miss Tidy, a graduate who had only recently joined the corporation and knew little about Horrormycin and even less about statistics. She was terrified of Dr Climber and soon learnt that he did not like being bothered with trivial queries, even on the rare occasions when he was in his office, so she kept them to herself and grew increasingly pale and thin in her solitary labours, and resolved to escape back to the happier land of Academia as soon as she could.

Dr Climber realised that a publication would enhance his reputation, and had grown to despise the snivelling Miss Tidy, so he hired Ms Literate from the Ritemmup Agency for this task. However, Dr Climber was a busy man, and the agency offices happened to be on his way to the golf course, so he simply flung the report at Ms Literate, along with a bag of gold, and demanded that she should produce a draft by the end of the week. He zoomed away on his corporate charger and soon was far too many leagues away to hear her plaintive wailing about identifying authors and journals.

As the conference season was approaching, Dr Donothing, who had failed to recruit a single patient to the study, sent smoke signals to Dr Climber, indicating that a trip to Costlyville would be most acceptable. Dr Climber was happy to agree (as he had also heard good reports about the Costlyville golf courses) but suggested his old friend Professor Regionale should be an author, as he had recruited one patient to the study, lived near Costlyville and might introduce him to the best golf club. Sadly, the smoke signals took a long time to reach Dr Climber and, by the time he replied, the deadline for submitting abstracts had passed, but this meant that the three men could enjoy the meeting (and the golf courses) without the tiresome distraction of making a presentation.

Meanwhile, in the cobweb-festooned corridors of Ritemmup, the paper progressed slowly and made many journeys back and forth to the caverns of marketing which lurked underneath Darke Towers. After the sixth round of comments, the owner of Ritemmup growled that the bag of gold would not cover any further embellishments and that it was time to get some authors for the paper. Dr Climber therefore sent the draft to Professor Regionale and also to Dr Seymour, a struggling young British doctor picked at random from the list of investigators because his name came after Professor Regionale's.

Honest Dr Seymour was surprised to receive the manuscript, since, despite recruiting several patients, he had never been told how the study had gone, so he asked for the original report. Dr Climber was glad to find somebody who took such an interest in the findings, but less delighted when Dr Seymour spotted a major problem with the analysis (caused by the inscrutable Dr Chi reading some tables from right to left, which had been overlooked by Miss Tidy). Fortunately, by this time, Mrs Countem had returned and, together with Dr Seymour, helped Ms Literate to prepare a totally revised version (but only after another bag of gold had been delivered to the agency).

The revised version was then sent to Dr Donothing, Professor Regionale and, at the suggestion of the marketing department, Dr Keen and Professor Igor, who lived in rich countries ravaged by disfiguring diseases that responded to Horrormycin. All except Dr Donothing added some comments and suggested changes to the paper, blissfully unaware of the original intentions of the study, and of the fact that the draft was now at least 1000 words over the limit for any journal. But Ms Literate applied her magic red quill pen, and produced another version. This was delivered, on a silver salver, to Dr Darke, the company's ageing and increasingly erratic founder, who invited the equally venerable and absent-minded Professor Importante to join the author list. Professor Importante could not remember if she had ever heard of this study, but she did not like to refuse her old friend. The paper descended once more into the vaults of the regulatory and legal gnomes and was finally submitted to the *Ivory Tower Journal of Impressive Results*.

The final list of authors was: Donothing, Regionale, Keen, Igor, Seymour, Climber and Importante. Somebody had found a yellowed parchment which stated that no more than one corporation employee could be included on any publication, so Mrs Countem was omitted in favour of the more persuasive and influential Dr Climber.

Meanwhile, unbeknown to Dr Climber, Dr Enthusiastikov, head of the Placebo Institute of Malpractica – which had recruited an unfeasibly large number of patients (many of whom were omitted from the main analysis since they failed to meet the inclusion criteria) – had analysed the data from his institute. He submitted a paper (in the Malpractican dialect) to the *Journal of Salami Science* (*JSS*) with himself as sole author and no mention of the Darke Corporation or the rest of the study because he had heard nothing from the Darke Corporation since the study ended, there was nothing in his contract to suggest he should not do this, and he was keen to enrich his CV with another publication.

By a strange stroke of fate, the *Ivory Tower Journal of Impressive Results* sent the paper to somebody who had already reviewed Dr Enthusiastikov's paper for the *JSS*, and she pointed out the similarities.

By this time, Dr Climber had lost all interest in Horrormycin and was devoting himself to Bustergut. He ignored Ms Literate's messages about the journal's concerns and concentrated on his golf handicap. Mrs Countem was disgruntled and unwilling to help, having been omitted from the author list and, as usual, Dr Donothing did nothing. A few months later, the Darke Corporation was swallowed up by Dragontooth Pharma, who stopped the development of Horrormycin, refused to give the Ritemmup Agency any more gold and sacked Mrs Countem as they disapproved of working mothers.

Dr Seymour was sorry that the study never got published, as he continued to see patients disfigured by infections that might have been cured by Horrormycin, but he was so busy administering other salves and potions that he soon forgot about it.

However, there is one magic formula guaranteed to stop papers from disappearing. It is called a 'publication strategy'. As with any form of magic, it can be used for both good and evil, and is a powerful force. Consult the rest of this book to discover how to achieve a good one!

Part two

A to Z of publication strategy

A

■ Abstracts

■ For conferences

Submission deadlines for abstracts to major conferences are non-negotiable. Organisers of smaller meetings occasionally extend their deadlines if they have not received as many abstracts as they hoped for, but you should never bank on this. If you have a really good reason why you cannot meet the deadline (e.g. your results will be available only a few days later) or you have good links with the organising committee it might be worth contacting the organisers well before the deadline to see if there is any flexibility. But, in most cases, you will need to plan carefully to ensure you meet the deadline.

Despite their brevity, a lot can go wrong with abstracts, especially those that are submitted electronically on behalf of other people.

Tips to avoid delays and nervous breakdowns when submitting abstracts

Check the conference website well in advance for requirements such as:

- having abstracts sponsored by a member of the organising association
- limiting the number of abstracts each member can submit or sponsor
- limiting the number of abstracts on which an individual can be listed as first author.

In addition, check practical requirements such as:

- word limit
- whether tables are permitted
- preferred structure/headings.

Find out what author details are required then obtain these well in advance. Details you might have forgotten could include:

- middle names/initials
- full postal address of institution
- telephone number (for presenting/first author)
- fax number (for presenting/first author)
- e-mail address (for all authors)

- membership number/name as it appears in the membership directory for sponsor
- authors' dates of birth (especially if they are eligible for 'young presenter' awards)
- any other obscure facts about the authors that you are unlikely to know (I recently heard of a conference website that required the authors' passport numbers).

Also check what other decisions you will need to make. Make sure you discuss these with all authors and key players:

- key words
- topic/area of presentation (often selected from a list of sessions)
- presentation preference (oral/poster).

As with any publication, allow sufficient time to get approval from all co-authors, your boss/institution and funding body, as appropriate.

Since an abstract is often the first publication to be developed from a research project, it is often the first document in which the authors are listed. A looming deadline is not conducive to rational and even-tempered discussion about author inclusion or order, so get this agreed well in advance (*see* **authorship** for guidance on this).

The principles of authorship used by journals generally apply to conference abstracts (although conference websites rarely bother to mention this). However, there is no absolute rule stating that the order of authors on an abstract must be identical to that on the final paper and it is acceptable to include local authors if they are presenting the findings at regional meetings or in different languages.

Electronic submission of abstracts via a conference abstract brings its own problems. Watch out for the following.

- The system used on the website to calculate the number of words will not necessarily produce the same figure as your software; be prepared to make last-minute adjustments if you are up to the word limit.
- Some websites will not accept unusual characters (e.g. Greek letters), symbols (e.g. ±), or foreign accents; consider using alternatives, e.g. mcg instead of µg, ae for German ä, etc.
- Even if websites appear to accept unusual characters, try to check their final appearance as they sometimes get garbled (e.g. Greek µ can turn into m with drastic consequences for drug doses).
- Increasing traffic as the deadline approaches may make conference websites slow to respond or collapse altogether. Aim to submit your abstract as early as possible to avoid the rush.

If you know you will have to submit an abstract close to the deadline and perhaps without time to contact the authors about last-minute queries it is a good idea to do a 'dummy submission'. Many websites only allow you to see all the pages (and therefore discover what information is required) once you have started a submission, so it makes sense to have a trial run going through all the pages just up to the actual submission. This will show you exactly what you need for the submission and should avoid last-minute hitches.

Try to agree the contents in good time with all the authors. Discussing the **key messages** of the research will be time well spent, since you can often only squeeze one or two major outcomes into an abstract.

Unlike papers, ethical rules about redundant publication do not apply. You may therefore split your findings over several abstracts (e.g. one on safety, one on efficacy, one on a sub-group analysis). You may also submit similar or identical abstracts to several meetings (unless a conference accepts only new data or holds the copyright of abstracts). In general, the largest (US and international) meetings will not accept findings that have been presented elsewhere. It therefore pays to plan your meetings carefully, if necessary reserving the first presentation for a large meeting, and using smaller, national or regional meetings for secondary presentations. Including trial registration numbers on abstracts (as recommended by CONSORT for Abstracts and GPP3) should make it clear when several presentations relate to the same study and help to link abstracts to full papers.

Abstracts submitted to meetings do not prevent later submissions of full reports to journals. However, *see* the sections on **prior publication** and **encore abstracts** for more details.

■ Of a paper

The abstract is a crucial part of the paper and, in many cases, the only part that gets read. This means it must be accurate, and it ought to be sufficiently interesting to entice your audience to read the rest of the paper. Some journal editors perform their initial screening by reading only the abstract. An announcement in *The BMJ* contained the advice: 'Please get the abstract right, because we may use it alone to assess your paper'.

The easiest time to write the abstract is after you have written the rest of the paper. Check the journal's instructions for word limits and structure. If the journal does not stipulate a structure consider using headings as they improve readability.

Abstract headings are usually similar to those in the main body of the text, i.e. Introduction (or Background, or Objectives), Methods, Results, Conclusion.

Most journals limit the size of abstracts and indexing services may truncate abstracts. For example, **Medline** used to cut abstracts off after 250 words even if a longer version appeared in the journal. However, the Medline limit is now 10 000 characters (or about 1000 words) so, in practice, this isn't usually a problem. Try to follow CONSORT for Abstracts, which provides a useful checklist on the content.

Although it may be tempting to leave writing the abstract until a late draft of the paper, do not leave it too late. All authors should have sufficient time to comment on this important section of the paper. However, remember to update the abstract whenever other parts of the paper are changed. The abstract should never contain findings that do not appear in the main text. Round up numbers consistently so that figures in the main text and abstract are identical. If a figure can sensibly be rounded up in the abstract, consider rounding it up elsewhere. Strings of decimal places reduce readability and often do not add anything meaningful.

Groves T and Abbasi K (2004) Screening research papers by reading abstracts. *BMJ*. **329**: 470–1.

Hopewell S, Clarke M, Moher D *et al.* (2008) CONSORT for reporting randomised trials in journal and conference abstracts. *Lancet*. **371**: 281–3.

■ Acceptance rates

■ Journals

These range from 5% to 85% and should therefore be a major factor when select-ing a target journal. Well-known general journals such as *The Lancet* and *The New England Journal of Medicine* (*NEJM*) reject over 90% of the papers they receive, while new, electronic journals or those operating a 'bias to publish' reject only around 15%. Some journals publish their acceptance statistics each year and others give some idea of this on their websites or in their 'Instructions to authors'. If you can-not find the precise figure, assume:

- prestigious general journals 5–20%
- prestigious specialist journals 10–30%
- other specialist journals 30–50%
- new titles, obscure journals 40–70%
- non-selective 'bias to publish' journals 70–90%.

Submitting to a journal with a frighteningly low acceptance rate may not be a bad strategy, but you should always have a **back-up plan** in case you are rejected, and you should think about what effects rejection might have on your timetable (*see* **acceptance times** and **rejection**).

■ Meetings

These are generally much higher than for journals; 50–70% is not uncommon. However, unlike journals many conferences do not publicise their acceptance rates so they can be hard to ascertain. Since you may submit similar abstracts to several meetings, their acceptance rates need not concern you as much as journals when planning a publication strategy.

■ Acceptance times

The time from submission to acceptance varies enormously between journals so this will be an important criterion for selection if speed is important to you. Many journals give some idea of decision times in their 'Instructions to authors', but bear in mind that these may be averages or even optimistic targets (beware of phrases such as 'we aim to give a decision in four weeks …'). Some helpful journals publish their actual performance statistics each year.[1] Others give information about acceptance times by publishing submission and acceptance dates on each article. In other cases, ask a colleague who has submitted something to the journal in the last few years.

Bear in mind that time to acceptance is often longer than time to rejection, especially in journals that reject a large proportion of papers after in-house review. Time to acceptance also includes the time taken by authors to respond to reviewers' comments (which journal editors delight in reminding us can be lengthy) and time for additional rounds of review.

1 For example, Bauchner H, Fontanarosa PB and Golub RM (2015) To *JAMA* authors, peer reviewers, and readers – thank you. *JAMA*. **313**: 675–6.

See also **rejection** and Chapter 3 'How long will it take?' (pp. 13–17).

■ Access to data

Good Publication Practice recommends that sponsors should 'provide authors with access to all of the study information necessary to prepare the publication or presentation (e.g., protocol, statistical analysis plan, study report) before writing begins, allow relevant access to anonymized patient-level data, and provide reasonable additional analyses in support of the publication upon request'. This responsibility should be set out in the **publication agreement**. The 2015 revision (GPP3) extends this recommendation and suggests that sponsors should also 'grant access to patient-level data to qualified researchers on request' while noting that such reports 'should be redacted to protect patient confidentiality.'

See also **ownership of data**.

■ Accountability of authors

The 2013 update of the ICMJE authorship guidelines added a fourth criterion relating to accountability. The *Nature* journals (which set their own authorship guidelines rather than following the ICMJE) have also stressed the importance of all authors taking accountability for the work. Sadly, the ICMJE never explains or expands on its pronouncements, so authors (and those setting authorship guidelines for organisations) have to work out for themselves what accountability really means.

Here's my interpretation. I think it's significant that ICMJE used the term 'accountability' rather than 'responsibility'. It would be unreasonable to expect authors to take responsibility for something done by somebody else, in another centre, and quite possibly on another continent. You can't stand over your colleagues and check each measurement or calculation they make. However, if, at any stage after submitting the manuscript to the journal (or after publication), somebody spots a potential problem or error it's not good enough simply to say, 'It's not my problem – I didn't do that bit.' I think what the editors mean by accountability is that all authors agree that they will cooperate (and, if necessary chase their co-authors) to get to the bottom of any problem and make sure it is sorted out even if the problem relates to part of the work they weren't directly involved with.

My guess is that the new criterion arose because editors were fed up with the author most strongly suspected of error or misconduct not responding, or being evasive, while all the other authors (and their institutions) said, 'It's not my problem – I didn't do that bit.' But, as I say, these are just my interpretations. However you interpret the ICMJE criterion, it highlights an important point that authorship brings both credit and accountability, so be careful what you put your name to.

■ Acknowledgements

■ People

Some journals, for example *JAMA* and *Annals of Internal Medicine*, require the corresponding author to state that written confirmation has been received from everybody mentioned in the acknowledgements. GPP3 also recommends that those named in the acknowledgements should review the wording and give written permission for being included. It is therefore a good idea to include the acknowledgements in an early draft so that you are not delayed by gathering the confirmations. Even if journals do not require written confirmation it is only polite to inform anybody you plan to acknowledge and you should respect their request if they prefer not to be named. Use the acknowledgements section to thank people who have helped the project but do not merit authorship, such as investigators outside the writing group, study nurses, data monitors and medical writers or author's editors.

Check journal instructions to see what roles can be acknowledged. Although acknowledgements are generally used to record the contributions of medical writers who do not fulfil the **International Committee of Medical Journal Editors' (ICMJE)** criteria for authorship, a few journals, notably *Neurology*, insist that 'professional writers employed by pharmaceutical companies ... who have drafted or revised the intellectual content of the paper must be included as authors'.

■ Funding

The source of funding or support for research (including writing assistance) should always be described. Many journals include funding details in the acknowledgements section, but some put this information in a footnote on the title page, or in the methods (*see* **sponsor, role of** for more details). It is good practice to include some kind of **trial identifier**, such as a trial registration number. Identifying the trial helps people preparing systematic reviews and may discourage **redundant publication**. Members of the **ICMJE** have required trial registration as a condition for publication in their journals since July 2005 and many other journals have followed their lead.

De Angelis C, Drazen JM, Frizelle FA *et al.* (2004) Clinical trial registration: a statement from the International Committee of Medical Journal Editors. *Lancet.* **364**: 911–12.

Wager E (2004) The need for trial identifiers. *Curr Med Res Opin.* **20**: 203–6.

■ Advertising departments

If you want detailed information about who reads a journal and where these readers work, the best source is the advertising department (if the journal has one). This department uses such information to persuade customers to place advertisements in the journal. If the journal does not carry display advertisements, you could try contacting the editorial office or subscriptions department, but they may not have the information in such detail or it may be difficult to find the correct person to speak to.

■ Affiliations; *see authors' affiliations*

■ American Medical Writers Association (AMWA)

This organisation produces a code of ethics for medical writers[1] and has issued a position statement on their involvement with publications.[2] Its European sister organisation the **European Medical Writers Association** (EMWA) has also produced a statement.[3]

1 www.amwa.org/amwa_ethics

2 www.amwa.org/position_statement

3 Jacobs A and Wager E (2005) European Medical Writers Association (EMWA) guidelines on the role of medical writers in developing peer-reviewed publications. *Curr Med Res Opin.* **21**: 317–22. Available at www.emwa.org/documents/about_us/EMWA guidelines.pdf

■ Anonymous reviewers

Most journals do not disclose the identity of reviewers to authors. Anonymity is supposed to enable reviewers to speak their mind without fearing the consequences. Its supporters claim that anonymity overcomes the problem of junior scientists being unwilling to criticise the work of more senior researchers for fear of damaging their careers. However, a few journals have challenged this idea and now practise 'open reviewing', arguing that it is fairer if authors know the identity of their reviewers. *The BMJ* studied the effects of open review before adopting it. The studies found that open review was feasible (i.e. only a tiny proportion of reviewers refused to sign) but had little discernible effect on review quality or tone. This should reassure those who feared that reviewers would be reluctant to criticise work if they knew their name would be revealed to authors. However, it does not support the opposing view that open review would produce more detailed, or more courteous, reviews.

Even if the journal does not reveal reviewers' names, many authors think they can guess their reviewers' identity, but they are often wrong.[1] It is therefore unwise to bear a lifelong grudge against somebody you suspect of reviewing your work harshly; it was probably somebody else.

Even if you know who has reviewed your paper, you should not contact the reviewers directly to discuss (or dispute) their suggestions, even if that seems the simplest way to resolve a disagreement. You should always address reviewers' comments via the editor.

Some journals ask authors to suggest potential reviewers, or allow them to indicate if there is anybody they do not want as a reviewer (*see* **reviewer choice**). However, unless the journal practises open review you may never know if your suggestions were adopted.

Some journals take anonymity one stage further by trying to mask the authors' identity – *see* **blinded (masked) review** for more details.

1 Wesseley S, Brugha T, Cowen P *et al.* (1996) Do authors know who refereed their paper? A questionnaire survey. *BMJ.* **313**: 1185.

■ Appeals

A rejection is always disappointing, and fighting it may be a natural reaction, but it is usually better to swallow your pride and switch to your **back-up plan**. However, there are a few circumstances when it may be worth appealing a decision. One is when you receive at least one favourable review but the journal editor seems to be swayed by a single negative review. If you can give objective reasons why the negative reviewer is wrong, or demonstrates bias, it may be worth sending a carefully worded letter to the editor. Unless you know the editor well, you should not telephone as most editors will consider only written appeals. Before you appeal, look carefully at the editor's letter for clues about the reason for rejection. If the editor indicates that your submission is not suited to the journal there is little point in appealing, even if some of the reviewers' comments are favourable.

The BMJ's instructions to contributors advise: 'Appeals clarifying and revising specific parts of the manuscript, for instance the analysis of original data, tend to succeed much more often than appeals against essentially editorial decisions where we did not think *The BMJ* was the right journal for the article because it did not fit well with *The BMJ*'s readers' needs and interests.' *The BMJ* also points out that 'we can consider only one appeal per manuscript. We have found that prolonged negotiation over rejected papers are usually unsatisfactory for both authors and editors.'[1]

If you feel that a journal has mistreated you in some way, other than by failing to recognise the brilliance of your work, you should write to the editor or, if the journal has one, the **ombudsman/ombudsperson**. Alerting the editor to your grievance may not undo the damage but it might help other authors by preventing future problems, and getting the matter off your chest may be therapeutic. Many journals track reviewer performance so a letter from an author might encourage the editor to avoid that reviewer in future.

The **Committee on Publication Ethics (COPE)** considers cases brought by journal editors which may involve misconduct by authors or reviewers. However, COPE does not consider cases from aggrieved authors about editorial decisions. If you feel you have not got a satisfactory response from the editor, you could approach the journal's governing body, especially if this is an academic society, or the publisher. The **World Association of Medical Editors (WAME)** has an ethics committee that considers cases from members, not all of whom are journal editors, so this might offer a possible avenue for complaint if you feel you have been badly treated.

Whatever you do, make sure you do not spend so much energy on your grievances and appeals that you have none left to implement your **back-up plan**.

1 www.bmj.com/about-bmj/resources-authors/article-submission/appeals

■ Approval

Final approval of the version to be published is one of the four criteria for **authorship** promoted by the International Committee of Medical Journal Editors. However, exceptions are usually made if an author dies (or becomes incapacitated) at a late stage in the publication process. **Good Publication Practice** (GPP3) emphasises that 'the authors are responsible for all final decisions on publication content, for final approval of the versions for submission, and of the version for publication or presentation'. GPP3 also notes that companies' commercial functions (i.e. their marketing departments) should not be involved in publication review or approval.

■ Article formats

Always check your target journal to see what types of articles it accepts. It is a surprisingly common mistake to identify a journal by its readership or impact factor and to ignore the fact that it simply never publishes the type of paper you have prepared.

Even if a journal publishes the type of article you have in mind, check whether it considers unsolicited manuscripts. Many journals publish only commissioned **editorials** and opinion pieces, so unsolicited ones can be hard to place. Others will not consider unsolicited review articles. The best strategy is to make an initial enquiry to the editor to see if you can interest him/her in your idea.

A few journals will not consider editorials or non-systematic reviews from authors with competing interests. Other, and to my mind more enlightened, journals regard transparency as the key and try to ensure that any potential **conflict of interest** is stated so that reviewers and readers can decide for themselves. Honesty is definitely the best policy – all authors should be prepared to disclose potential competing interests both financial and personal – but bear in mind that this might bar you from publishing certain types of articles in some journals.

■ Article processing charge (APC)

Most **Open Access journals** charge an APC. This is generally a set price per article (hence the name) and is charged *after* acceptance (not on submission) so you don't pay anything if your manuscript is rejected. Reputable journals will waive this fee for authors from low income countries and may waive or reduce fees for other authors whose research is unfunded. APCs have almost completely replaced the page charges levied by some (so-called pay journals) in the past.

A handful of journals also charge a **submission fee** – this is a much smaller amount than most APCs and is justified (by those that do it) by the costs of administering peer review and perhaps also as a deterrent against multiple submission and subsequent withdrawal (which, despite being outlawed, is apparently still a problem for some journals). While it may be reasonable to pay a small sum before your article is accepted, you should be very suspicious of journals that demand substantial sums on submission – they are likely to be **predatory journals**.

If your budget is limited, you should check the affordability of APCs and consider this when you select your target journal. Some (so-called **diamond**) **Open Access** journals do not charge APCs, and, of course, subscription journals don't charge authors unless they choose to make their article Open Access. It is also worth checking each target journal because APCs vary considerably even within the same publisher. Current (2015) APCs for major Open Access medical journals (or optional Open Access charges in major subscription journals) range from $1000 to $5000. *PeerJ* is an interesting exception, charging each author $99 for membership entitling him or her to publish one article per year for life (see https://peerj.com/pricing/).

■ Artwork; *see* figure legends; figures; graphs

■ Authors' affiliations

Authors' affiliations at the time they did the study should be listed on publications (even if they have moved). This helps readers understand where the work was done and credits the institutions. If authors have changed jobs since the research was done you should also include their current affiliation (this is often shown as a footnote). Ask all authors to check their details on the very first draft they see; do not wait until just before submission. Check with your institution for the correct way of naming it. If in doubt, check your payslip or headed notepaper to find the formal name of your employer. For example, for UK National Health Service (NHS) hospitals this is usually the name of the trust, rather than the more familiar name of a single hospital or clinic.

■ Authorship

The authorship of publications can cause many headaches. The two important rules are to:

- be familiar with recognised authorship criteria, for example those from the **International Committee of Medical Journal Editors (ICMJE)**
- discuss authorship early in the research process.

The ICMJE states that authors should be able to take public responsibility for the research and the publication. This normally involves contributing to study design or interpretation, as well as playing an active part in developing the publication and approving the final version.

The Medical Publishing Insights and Practices (MPIP) initiative has produced a helpful five-step framework for determining the authorship of company-sponsored research projects.[1] MPIP recommends establishing an authorship working group, defining substantial contributions and documenting contributions during the trial. It then becomes simpler to determine who has made a substantial contribution and check that authors meet other criteria such as involvement with the publication.

Some journals have abandoned the traditional author **by-line** for the **contributorship** system where individuals' contributions to the research are listed. Check which system your **target journal** uses. Also consult the sections on the **writing group, number of authors** and **order of authors**. To understand problems to avoid, *see* **ghost author(s)** and **guest authors/gift authorship** and read the tale of 'Dr Seymour and the disappearing paper' (pp. 23–5).

The ICMJE Recommendations relate to journal articles and there are few explicit guidelines on authorship for conference abstracts. **Good Publication Practice (GPP3)** is an exception, advising: 'The same authorship criteria used for journal publications (e.g., ICMJE) should be used for congress presentations … Encore presentations should usually have the same authorship as the original presentation. However, authorship of encore presentations at national or local meetings may differ slightly (e.g., to enable presentation in the appropriate language in situations where the congress does not allow nonauthor presenters), provided all original authors agree.'

For further reading try:

Albert T and Wager E (2003) How to handle authorship disputes: a guide for new researchers. *COPE Report 2003*. Committee on Publication Ethics, London. pp. 32–4. http://publicationethics.org/files/2003pdf12_0.pdf

1 Marusic A, Hren D, Mansi B *et al.* (2014) Five-step authorship framework to improve transparency in disclosing contributors to industry-sponsored clinical trial publications. *BMC Medicine.* **12**: 197.

B

■ Back-up plan

Selecting a **target journal** is not always easy because the **key players** may have different aims and expectations. For example, speed of publication may be the most important criterion for one person, while journal **impact factor** may be more important to another.

Since many journals have high rejection rates, and since it can take time to get agreement about the target journal, it is always a good idea to have a back-up plan and to select a second journal in case your paper is rejected by the first. If you do not select the second journal at the same time as the first you may miss an opportunity for discussion and waste a lot of time. A rejection is always unwelcome and, even if it is not entirely unexpected, it often leads to loss of motivation and momentum and thus further delay.

Choosing a second target journal may also help to meet varied expectations among authors. For example, if some authors are keen to aim for a prestigious journal, while others are more concerned about rapid publication, you might agree to submit first to a prestigious journal that uses **in-house review** and therefore has short rejection times, but agree to submit to a less prestigious journal with a greater chance of acceptance, and/or reasonably rapid publication, if your paper is rejected by the first.

■ Beall's list

This refers to the splendidly titled 'Beall's list: potential, possible, or probable predatory scholarly open-access journals'. This excellent resource is produced by University of Colorado Denver librarian Jeffrey Beall, who has launched a bold, one-man campaign against **predatory publishers**. If you ever doubt a journal's (or publisher's) credentials, check 'Beall's list' (at http://scholarlyoa.com/publishers/). To keep up to date you can subscribe to his blog and updates.

While it doesn't take long for more experienced authors and publication professionals to check a journal's website and publication record to see if it is reputable, a quick check of 'Beall's list' saves you the trouble. The resource is especially helpful for less seasoned researchers, particularly non-native English speakers, who may not spot the typos and odd wording that usually bedevil such websites and spam invitations from predators, which often serve as a useful alert to other authors. (My favourite was a website that announced in large letters that the journal checked for 'Palgiarism [sic]'.) Beall has also highlighted cases in which reputable journals have been hijacked by predatory clone websites which might fool anybody but, thankfully, are relatively rare (*see* **cloned journals**).

For more information *see* **predatory publishers**.

■ Bias

Scientists and clinicians are expected to have opinions about what their findings mean but they are also expected to present results fairly and responsibly. As with many ethical questions it is hard to provide a working definition of bias but the following examples of biased reporting give ideas about what to avoid.

Examples of reporting bias

- Presenting secondary or post hoc analyses as if they were the primary outcomes of a study if the primary outcomes did not turn out as you had hoped.
- 'Cherry picking' the most favourable outcomes or test results and omitting others that do not fit your hypothesis (e.g. reporting 6-month efficacy data but omitting 12-month results because they do not reach statistical significance, or reporting results of one rating scale but not another).
- Omitting adverse events or clumping them into meaningless categories (e.g. not detailing the number of deaths but including these among all serious adverse events).
- Failing to describe a study population adequately if some special features of this population might affect the results (e.g. reporting treatment preference without mentioning that patients had previously failed on another therapy).

■ Bibliographic software

Anybody who writes more than a couple of articles should consider investing in bibliographic software. Several brands are available, both commercial (e.g. EndNote and Reference Manager) and free (e.g. Mendeley). Using such software allows writers to organise reference sources and greatly reduces the hassle of producing reference lists that meet journal formatting requirements. Some systems even create a searchable library of downloaded PDFs or abstracts which is a bonus. These packages also allow you to download citation details directly from online sources such as Medline which not only saves you from tedious typing but also reduces the risk of errors in your references. Once you have created your library, the software allows you to switch formats (e.g. from numbered Vancouver style to author-date format) and most come preloaded with formats for masses of journals so there is no need for fine-tuning. Reference libraries may also be shared (e.g. between authors, within a company, or between authors and a professional writer) and most are compatible with each other, allowing import, export and further time savings.

While reference software is a wonderful tool for writers, publishers' attitudes to it vary. Some publishers encourage authors to use certain packages,[1] and may even offer reduced article processing charges to those that do, because their typesetting is set up to recognise the codes used by the software. Other publishers warn that the codes used by bibliographic software (which link manuscripts with the writer's reference libraries) may upset their typesetting processes and should therefore be stripped out before submission. As ever, the rule is to check your target journal's instructions carefully before submission (as I have mentioned before and will probably say again …).

1 BioMed Central (n.d.) Useful tools. www.biomedcentral.com/authors/authortools

■ 'Big Five'

- *Annals of Internal Medicine*
- *The BMJ* (*British Medical Journal*)
- *JAMA* (*The Journal of the American Medical Association*)
- *The Lancet*
- *The New England Journal of Medicine* (*NEJM*)

are sometimes known, informally, as the 'Big Five'. All but *Annals* are weekly, and they all have large subscription bases. They are all represented on the **International Committee of Medical Journal Editors** (**ICMJE**, or Vancouver Group) and have been influential in developing peer-review research and policy. Many studies of peer-review practices have focused on the Big Five, which is a pity, since, although they are undoubtedly influential, they are also atypical. Unlike smaller journals run by academic societies, the Big Five have full-time editors and large numbers of editorial staff. This means they reject up to 50% of submissions after internal review. They also tend to invest quite heavily in **technical editing**, so, if your paper is accepted, you can expect it to be knocked pretty firmly into **house style**. The Big Five is a purely subjective grouping and some of the larger specialty journals (such as *Circulation* and *Neurology*) operate in similar ways. However, such big journals do operate differently from those with part-time, academic editors, and you should bear this in mind when dealing with them.

■ BioMed Central

A series of electronic **Open Access journals**. They have some innovative features including open peer review, publishing reviewers' comments alongside papers and requiring authors to suggest potential reviewers. They also require that all randomised trials be entered into a trial register or given a unique **ISRCTN (International Standard Randomised Controlled Trial Number)** identifier. Not to be confused with **PubMed Central**.

See www.biomedcentral.com

■ Blinded (masked) review

Several studies have attempted to test whether it matters if reviewers know the identity of the authors. Overall, the results are inconclusive, with some studies showing an effect and others not. The idea behind blinded review is that reviewers may be prejudiced by the authors' prestige, or lack of it. One study examined this by sending two versions of the same paper to several reviewers. In one version, the authors were from prestigious institutions, while in the second version the authors came from a fictitious (and unimpressive-sounding) centre. Reviewers apparently demonstrated institutional bias by criticising the paper from the prestigious institution less harshly. However, other studies have shown the opposite effect, with well-known authors receiving tougher reviews than junior scientists. Studies have also shown that it is difficult to mask authors' identities effectively because authors tend to cite their own work and reviewers often recognise researchers in their own field.

As an author the only choice you have about whether your identity will be revealed to the reviewer, or whether the journal will reveal the reviewers' identity to you, is your choice of target journal (*see* **anonymous reviewers** for more details). If you feel strongly about this you may be able to discover the journal's methods in the 'Instructions to authors' guidance notes; but don't bank on it.

If you choose a journal that uses blinded review, try to facilitate this by putting all the author details on a separate title page and making sure author names do not appear in the filename or as a header or footer. For obvious reasons ophthalmology journals prefer the term 'masked' to 'blinded'.

■ Blogs

There has been an explosion in the number of channels available for communicating about science in the last 10 years and blogs are perhaps the most obvious. Many researchers have their own blogs while others contribute to group blogs or discussion forums in which they discuss topics related to their work. Such ponderings are obviously unregulated, un-peer reviewed and un-indexed, so they should not be the main venue for publishing original research, but authors and publication planners might consider how they fit into an overall communication strategy.

Most biomedical journals follow the ICMJE guidelines and will not consider work that has already been published. So, the question is whether mentioning something on a blog constitutes 'prior publication'. BioMed Central has published helpful guidelines on redundant publication for its journals[1] which, unlike the guidance from many other journals (which often read as if they were written in the 19th century), includes things like blogs and wikis. According to BioMed Central (and, of course, this may not apply to other publishers) 'data posted and discussion on wikis, blogs, electronic online notebooks, [and] networking websites' may be included in a journal article 'at the Editor(s)' discretion' and the publisher recommends contacting the journal's editorial office for more information.

While it may be risky to reveal your findings on a blog before you have published them in a journal, what about discussing them after publication? So long as you respect copyright (which will, of course, depend on where you publish) journals are generally very happy for authors to discuss their published work via blogs and other informal channels and there is even some evidence that this, along with other **social media** use, may increase the citation or download rate.

1 BioMed Central. Generally permissible and non-permissible forms of duplicate/overlapping publication. www.biomedcentral.com/about/duplicatepublication#table1

See also **personal websites** and **social media**.

■ Board of Editors in the Life Sciences (BELS)

A certification scheme, established in 1991, to evaluate the proficiency of manuscript editors in the life sciences. Editors who have passed the exam may use the letters BELS after their name. Some medical writers who also offer editing services may have this qualification, but a more relevant one to look out for is probably the **Certified Medical Publication Professional (CMPP)** which focuses on publication planning and preparation.

www.bels.org/

◾ Books

Primary publications of research should appear in peer-reviewed journals rather than books because journal articles generally take less time to be published and are searchable via indexing and abstracting systems. However, book chapters often provide useful subject reviews and may provide greater freedom in terms of length, scope and format than journals. A book is an excellent format if your aim is primarily to educate or entertain your readers. I hope that this one succeeds in doing a little of both.

◾ Brief

If you are working with a professional medical writer, the quality of their work, and the likelihood that it will please the authors, is directly related to the quality of the brief. Despite possessing many other superhuman qualities (such as writing ability and detailed knowledge of reporting guidelines), medical writers are not telepathic so it is essential that authors explain their needs and expectations clearly to the writer (or agency) at the outset (e.g. when an outline is being prepared). Even if the writer is armed with a copy of the study protocol, statistical tables, a clinical study report and the instructions from the target journal, it is essential that the authors agree among themselves, and communicate to the writer, the focus and aim of the publication. This will depend on the **key message** and **target audience**. Particular attention should be given to the introduction and discussion sections and usually also to the clinical interpretation of the findings (since medical writers are generally not clinical specialists).

Writers should not be embarrassed to question a brief if anything is unclear or to admit that they don't understand the authors' requests. Authors should view such exchanges as signs of a conscientious writer, keen to do a good job, rather than admissions of weakness. Nobody should be expected to put up with woolly briefs.

◾ By-line

Despite widespread endorsement of the **International Committee of Medical Journal Editors' (ICMJE)** guidelines, journal policies on authorship do vary. *See* **authorship** and **contributorship (vs. authorship)** for more detailed discussions of these concepts. Before the late 1990s, journals simply listed authors and their affiliations. This listing was equivalent to the by-line in a newspaper, which tells readers who an article is by. However, some journals now publish details of who did what. This list of contributors usually appears separately from the list of authors and so, in theory, it is possible for the contributor list to be different from the by-line. Further variation in practice occurs in how journals regard group names. Some will permit the formula 'Crank & Bloggs on behalf of the Whizzo Study Group' without the entire study group being listed, and without all the individual members of the study group fulfilling the journal's authorship criteria. However, other journals make a stricter interpretation of the by-line and insist that all members of a group are listed (for example in a footnote) and that all members meet authorship criteria.

Just to make things more confusing, some journals also include a separate listing of **collaborators**, who are subtly different from **contributors** and are now recognised in Medline.

For more information *see* **names** and **group authorship**.

C

■ Certified Medical Publication Professional (CMPP)

The **International Society for Medical Publication Professionals (ISMPP)** runs a certification scheme by which medical writers and publication planners can demonstrate their competence and, in particular, their knowledge of publication guidelines. Those who have passed an exam (which consists of 150 multiple-choice questions) are entitled to use the initials CMPP after their name. The accreditation lasts for 5 years, after which you must either pass the exam again or obtain educational credits by attending conferences and training to retain it. If you are considering working with a medical writer you might ask whether the person has passed this qualification. If you are selecting an agency to undertake publication work, you should ask whether it requires or encourages its staff to do so. However, ISMPP currently charges $495 to members and $690 to non-members to take the exam, which may deter freelancers and very small companies, and the scheme was only started in 2009, so some experienced writers, who already have a good customer base, may not feel it is worth doing. Therefore, lack of CMPP should not be taken to mean that the writer or agency is no good. However, the fact that somebody has obtained this certification suggests a high level of professionalism and an understanding of current publication guidelines, which has to be a good thing.

If you are reading this book in preparation for the CMPP exam I hope you find it helpful and wish you the best of luck!

See also **Board of Editors in the Life Sciences (BELS)**.

■ Checklists

Some journals include a checklist for submission within their 'Instructions to contributors'. What you need to submit depends on the journal. If your target journal provides a checklist, then follow it. If it does not, consider the following:

- **covering letter** – this should include a statement that the work is original and is not being considered for publication elsewhere
- authors' signatures/author declaration – stating that they have contributed to the publication and approved its submission
- authors' declarations of competing interests/financial support
- **copyright** transfer document – some journals require authors to relinquish copyright to the publisher – usually the corresponding author has to sign this
- authorisation from people mentioned in the **acknowledgements** or quoted as **personal communications**
- evidence that references cited as being 'in press' have been accepted for publication
- **permissions** to reproduce figures or tables from other publications
- consent from patients to publish personal details, e.g. in case studies.

■ ClinicalTrials.gov

This is a trial register sponsored by the United States National Library of Medicine. For more details look at www.clinicaltrials.gov. In September 2004 the **International Committee of Medical Journal Editors** announced that **trial registration** would be a condition for publication in their journals after July 2005.[1] At that time, only ClinicalTrials.gov met the editors' criteria but, since then, ICMJE has recognised other registers.

A US law, passed in 2007, made registration in ClinicalTrials.gov compulsory for most clinical trials. *See* **FDAAA** for more details. This Act also required study results to be posted on ClinicalTrials.gov so it has become a results repository as well as a trial register. Not to be confused with www.clinicaltrialresults.org (a sort of wiki for results, set up by researchers) or www.clinicalstudyresults.org (a results website run by **Pharmaceutical Research and Manufacturers of America (PhRMA)**.

1   De Angelis C, Drazen JM, Frizelle FA *et al.* (2004) Clinical trial registration: a statement from the International Committee of Medical Journal Editors. *Lancet.* **364**: 911–12.

■ Cloned journals

Another new phenomenon for authors to worry about (which has arisen since I wrote the second edition of this book). A few **predatory publishers**, not content with trying to lure authors with journal titles that are confusingly similar to existing, reputable journals, have hijacked genuine journals and produced predatory clone websites. While it is relatively easy to spot many predator journals because of amateurish or unconvincing websites, cloned or hijacked journals are harder to spot, although in most cases there are clues, such as a French language journal that suddenly started accepting articles in English, or a journal that suddenly broadened its scope from philosophy to science.

Fortunately, such scams are relatively rare in medicine (most of the ones on Beall's listing are biology journals), and much less common than the other type of predator journal, but it's as well to know about them so you won't be fooled. If in doubt, check Jeffrey Beall's blog (he has a specific list of hijacked journals at http://scholarlyoa.com/other-pages/hijacked-journals/), or try to access a journal via a recognised publisher or academic society whose website you can trust.

■ Co-authors

If you are having trouble deciding who your co-authors should be, consult the sections on **authorship**, **order of authors** and **number of authors**.

Remember to involve all authors as fully as possible when developing a publication plan and to consult them over all decisions, however minor. People can have strong feelings about the most unexpected aspects of publication strategy (*see* **expectations**). It is therefore remarkably easy for co-authors to fall out with or irritate each other.

If you develop a tough hide yourself, but assume that everybody else is likely to be injured by the slightest snub, you should survive, and might even live to work together on future projects. *See* **nitpickers** for hints on dealing with this particular species of co-author.

Remember that treating co-authors respectfully does not mean that you should be vague about what you want them to do. Clarity of communication is important, and it is always good to be explicit about deadlines and other requirements.

On a practical point, try to gather all the information you will need about your co-authors as early as possible. This may include full **names**, **affiliations**, qualifications, contact details, membership of relevant organisations (if this is required to submit an abstract) and statements on **competing interests**.

■ Collaborators

Just when you thought you understood the subtle distinctions between authors, contributors and acknowledgees (and the different definitions of these used by various journals), here comes another category: collaborators. This term has been available as a field in Medline since 2008. According to the Medline website 'when a group name is included as an author, the respective group member names appearing in the article will be acknowledged as collaborators but not associated with authorship'.

The International Committee of Medical Journal Editors advises: 'When submitting a manuscript authored by a group, the corresponding author should specify the group name if one exists, and clearly identify the group members who can take credit and responsibility for the work as authors. The byline of the article identifies who is directly responsible for the manuscript, and MEDLINE lists as authors whichever names appear on the byline. If the byline includes a group name, MEDLINE will list the names of individual group members who are authors or who are collaborators, sometimes called non-author contributors, if there is a note associated with the byline clearly stating that the individual names are elsewhere in the paper and whether those names are authors or collaborators.'

Knecht LWS and Nahin AM (2008) Study collaborators included in MEDLINE®/PubMed®. *NLM Tech Bull*. **March–April**: e2.

■ Committee on Publication Ethics (COPE)

COPE was established by journal editors to provide help with ethical issues. The committee discusses cases anonymously and then offers advice. COPE considers troublesome cases from editors but does not accept complaints from aggrieved authors. The COPE website contains much useful information on publication ethics; for example, how journals respond to cases of possible misconduct. See www.publicationethics.org.

■ Competing interest; *see* conflict of interest

■ Conditional acceptance

This is the most common positive response you will receive from a journal. It does not mean that your submission has been accepted, but offers definite hope of acceptance if you can address the reviewers' concerns.

Some journals ask reviewers to indicate whether a submission should be accepted with minor modification or only after substantial revision. Most journals only give a conditional acceptance to the first category. If a major rewrite is required you will probably be invited to resubmit (which is a bit worse than a conditional acceptance but still better than a rejection).

However, even though the requested changes may be relatively minor, the conversion rate between conditional and full acceptance does vary between journals, so you must be realistic. Discovering the odds of making the leap from conditional to full acceptance requires a good understanding of your target journal's peer-review process.

Journals fall into five categories.

1. *Journals with a 'bias to publish' (sometimes called non-selective or 'mega-journals', e.g. PLOS One)*: expect authors to make a reasonable attempt to answer reviewers' questions, but then accept virtually all submissions from those that do.
2. *Academic journals in which the editor makes the final decision based on the referees' reports*: expect authors to address referees' concerns or give reasons why they

have not made any suggested changes, but probably accept most submissions that get favourable referees' reports without consulting the referees again.

3. *Academic journals that return the revised submission to the original reviewers*: in these journals your submission could be rejected if you cannot address all the reviewers' concerns.

4. *Journals that send the revised version to new or additional reviewers*: this can be extremely frustrating, since the new reviewer may suggest quite different changes from the original ones. This sometimes feels like entering another review round and it is difficult to predict the likelihood of full acceptance. This usually happens if the original reviewers say they don't want to see your article again or that it requires specialist review, most commonly by a statistician.

5. *Journals where the final decision is made by the editorial board or a committee*: a conditional acceptance from this type of journal has the lowest chance of turning into a full acceptance. For example, *The Lancet* accepts only about one-third of the papers that reach this stage, regardless of how thoroughly the authors have responded to the reviewers' comments. In effect, this committee stage represents a third hurdle for submissions. Not only does the submission have to fall within the scope of the journal (which is determined by in-house review), it also has to pass the scientific scrutiny of the reviewers (hurdle number two) and finally, to get published, it has to be one of the most interesting submissions reviewed by the committee that week (or month).

So, your chance of full acceptance after receiving a conditional acceptance ranges from around 30% to over 90%, depending on the journal. The trick is to understand your target journal and therefore understand where you stand.

Of course, there are also other factors that may affect whether a conditional acceptance turns into a full one. If you refuse to follow the reviewers' and editor's recommendations your chances will be reduced. And, in some cases, reviewers make suggestions that are impossible for you to meet, for example demanding data that you did not collect, or a further analysis that you are not prepared to do.

Remember that a conditional acceptance is not the same as a full acceptance, so you cannot cite your paper as being 'in press' until you get the final acceptance letter. Remember to build in time for responding to reviewers' comments, and possibly for a further round of review, if you are trying to work out how long the overall process to publication will take.

■ Conflict of interest / competing interest

The **International Committee of Medical Journal Editors (ICMJE)** defines conflict of interest as 'when professional judgment concerning a primary interest (such as … the validity of research) may be influenced by a secondary interest (such as financial gain)'. It also notes that perceptions of conflicts of interest are as important as actual ones. The **World Association of Medical Editors (WAME)** also emphasises the importance of perceptions about competing interests in its definition: 'Conflict of interest (COI) exists when there is a divergence between an individual's private interests (competing interests) and his or her responsibilities to scientific and publishing activities such that a reasonable observer might wonder if the individual's behavior or judgment was motivated by considerations of his or her competing interests'. Most journals now require authors (and reviewers) to declare their interests. Most concentrate on financial interests such as employment, consultancies, research funding and stock ownership but conflicts can occur for other reasons such as personal relationships and institutional loyalty or even religious or political beliefs. Some journals (and institutions such as the US Food and Drug Administration) have attempted to set thresholds for financial relationships, considering that owning half a dozen shares in a big company is different from owning half the company. But, in most cases, it is up to the author to decide what to declare. A good rule is to think of the most cynical person imaginable, who will impute a bad motive wherever possible, and to ask yourself what he or she might consider could have influenced the conduct or reporting of your research. Journal editors have paid increasing attention to competing interests after some highly publicised cases where authors tried to conceal their connections with research sponsors, such as tobacco companies. This led some journals (e.g. the *NEJM*) to attempt to prevent people with any competing interests from writing editorials and reviews. However, many journals found this unworkable, since the best qualified and most experienced people usually have some links with major research sponsors (which, for drugs and devices, usually means commercial companies), or simply have policies to encourage transparency. But check before you plan to write an editorial.

Over the years, journals have evolved their own standards and recommendations on disclosure thresholds. This led to a rather messy situation in which an author might be expected to disclose financial relationships over the life of a project for one journal, going back 3 years for another journal and 5 years in another – leading to apparent inconsistencies (and even cases in which authors who had simply followed a journal's rules were accused of covering up certain interests). In an attempt to impose uniformity, the ICMJE issued a uniform disclosure form in October 2009 (available at www.icmje.org/coi_disclosure.pdf). This is used by ICMJE member journals and some others.[1]

Gather information about all authors' competing interests as soon as possible (don't wait until just before submission). Some journals provide a tick list, others leave authors to devise their own wording for the declaration. Including a competing interest statement in an early draft gives authors a chance to read what co-authors have written and may jog memories about things that ought to be declared, or suggest helpful wording or ways to present this information accurately but concisely.

There is no excuse for attempting to conceal a conflict of interest, but research suggests that declarations can influence readers' perceptions of a publication. Editors at *The BMJ* sent two versions of a paper to 300 subscribers. The only difference between the versions was that one stated the authors were employed by a fictitious drug company, while the other stated that the authors had no competing interests. The 170 readers who responded were not only more sceptical about the version with the competing interest, rating it as less believable and less valid than the one with untainted authors, but they also rated it as less interesting and less relevant.[2]

Decisions about authorship of publications reporting research should never be influenced by considerations about competing interests. If a company employee merits authorship, he or she should be listed. However, if you are planning a letter to the editor or an editorial you might consider whether involving an author with a strong competing interest could lessen its impact in the eyes of sceptical readers.

1 Drazen JM, Van Der Weyden MB, Sahni P et al. (2009) Uniform format for disclosure of competing interests in ICMJE journals. *N Engl J Med*. **361**: 1896–7.

2 Chaudhry S, Schroter S, Smith R et al. (2002) Does declaration of competing interests affect readers' perceptions? A randomised trial. *BMJ*. **325**: 1391–2.

Gottlieb S (2002) *New England Journal* loosens its rules on conflict of interest. *BMJ*. **324**: 1474.

James A and Horton R (2003) *The Lancet's* policy on conflicts of interest. *Lancet*. **361**: 8–9.

Smith R (1998) Beyond conflict of interest. Transparency is the key. *BMJ*. **317**: 291–2.

■ Congress / conference choice

A quick scan of websites listing medical congresses shows a dizzying number, so how do you choose the right one(s) for presenting your work? Some of the factors you need to consider are essentially the same as for **target journals**, namely **target audience**, reputation and **acceptance rates**. In addition you need to consider the following.

- *Timing*:
  - — can you produce your abstract to meet the submission deadline?
  - — does the timing of the meeting suit your strategy (e.g. to coincide with a product launch, or to ensure no interference with the main publication)?
- *Location*: can you afford to attend (and, let's face it, is it somewhere you would like to go)? Will your institution/company let you attend? These days most companies not only have budgetary restrictions but may also have security considerations; even if these do not affect you directly they may affect other delegates, e.g. attendance at conferences in the Middle East, including Turkey, has dropped since 2001.
- *Cost*: as well as getting to the meeting, you need to budget for the conference fees, accommodation and the cost of producing a poster or slides.
- *Special requirements*: some meetings require abstracts to be sponsored by members of the organising society, or may restrict the number of abstracts each member can submit.

- *Congress accepting data that have been presented previously*: some major international and US meetings will accept only new data, but smaller meetings do not impose such restrictions. You should therefore aim to have the first presentation at a major (i.e. fussy) meeting and encores at smaller (less fussy) ones *not* vice versa. *See* **encore abstracts** for more details. Most meetings do not accept data that have already been published in full (i.e. as a journal article).

It is acceptable to submit essentially the same abstract to several meetings, especially if participants come from different specialties or regions. However, you should avoid submitting multiple abstracts to meetings that are likely to have widely overlapping audiences, since participants may not share your enthusiasm for your research and probably will not appreciate seeing your results several times.

For information about what conferences are taking place do an internet search or refer to one of the many websites that offer this information such as: www. emedevents.com or the Congress Resource Center on www.docguide.com/crc.

For information about specific conferences, check their websites and ask people who have attended previous meetings. Colleagues may be your only source of information about the reputation of meetings, since, unlike journals, there are no **impact factors**. You could also search professional or topic-focused web-based discussion sites for opinions about what meetings are really like. Colleagues may also be the best source of information about acceptance rates, since congresses rarely publish these. However, since, unlike journals, you can submit abstracts to several meetings at once, the acceptance rates are less crucial than for journals. Information about conferences is also commercially available from communication agencies or specialist providers such as **DataVision** and **PubStrat**.

■ Consolidated Health Economic Evaluation Reporting Standards (CHEERS)

A guideline for reporting health economic studies, developed by the International Society for Pharmacoeconomics and Outcomes Research (ISPOR), presumably over a few drinks, in 2013. It has been endorsed by several journals and is worth checking if you are publishing this type of research.

www.ispor.org/taskforces/economicpubguidelines.asp

■ CONSORT

The CONSORT statement is an essential resource for anybody reporting results of randomised controlled trials. The recommendations were developed because published reports did not contain enough information for people preparing systematic reviews. The statement aims to be evidence based and it has been adopted by several hundred journals. Even if you are submitting a paper to a journal that has not formally adopted the CONSORT statement it is a good idea to follow it. The accompanying checklist is helpful, especially if you have not written this sort of paper before. The statement contains a lot of detail on reporting statistical methods and has a strong emphasis on robust randomisation and methods of minimising bias. It recommends that reports should include a figure (often called a CONSORT diagram) showing what happened to patients during a trial. Although they tend to be published only for more complex studies, preparing such a diagram can be a useful exercise and help to resolve queries about vanishing patients. Submitting a CONSORT diagram with your paper (even though you don't expect it will be published) may also show that you are aware of the guidelines and followed them when you wrote your report.

The statement is available at www.consort-statement.org or www.equator-network.org (which is a useful site containing links to many reporting guidelines).

■ CONSORT for Abstracts

A more recent addition to the CONSORT family is a checklist of items to include when reporting randomised trials in abstracts for conferences or journal articles. It recommends including a trial registration number and details about study funding. Some, but by no means all, of the journals that have adopted the main CONSORT statement have also adopted these guidelines, so check the instructions. Realising that journals like to do their own thing, CONSORT for Abstracts does not stipulate the format or headings that the abstract should contain, so you also need to check individual journal and conference requirements for these. Including all the items in the checklist should make your abstract more useful to readers (including reviewers and editors) so it makes sense to follow the guidance even if the journal or congress doesn't explicitly require it (but I'm biased, as I helped develop the guideline!).

Hopewell S, Clarke M, Moher D *et al.* (2008) CONSORT for reporting randomised trials in journal and conference abstracts. *Lancet.* **371**: 281–3.

■ Contact details

Journals require full contact details for the **corresponding author**. This usually means full postal address, telephone and fax numbers, and e-mail address. Remember to inform the journal if any details change after submission, otherwise your notification of acceptance or proofs may go astray. If you are not the corresponding author, try to obtain these details on an early draft. It is bothersome to have to delay submission because you forgot to get the corresponding author's fax number (and s/he is guaranteed to be away when you need this urgently).

■ Contracts

Research is rarely a solo exercise and large projects virtually always involve some sort of relationship between a sponsor/funder and the investigator(s). The nature of this relationship should be set out in an **investigators' agreement** or contract.

The contract is an excellent place to record decisions about the planned publication strategy, but, sadly, many sponsors ignore this opportunity or include only minimal details. Many problems with publications arise because sponsor and investigator have not discussed the strategy or have different **expectations** about it. Such problems get harder to resolve if they are left until the end of a project. It therefore makes sense to discuss publication plans at the earliest stage and to get agreement before the contract is signed.

Although it will not be possible to determine who will qualify as an author before the research has started, it should be possible to set out principles about how a **writing group** will be constituted. It is never too early to start discussing this.

Contracts should include something about data ownership and data access. If you feel a proposed contract is unduly restrictive, get advice from your boss and/or institution. **Good Publication Practice (GPP3)** states that companies should never attempt to **veto** publications, although they may, legitimately, 'review drafts in a timely manner to ensure accuracy, compliance with regulatory requirements, and protection of their intellectual property'. Some journals now ask authors to state whether they had free access to the data and how much control the sponsor had over the decision to publish.

Unfortunately there have been cases in which investigators signed restrictive contracts permitting sponsors to suppress a publication. In these cases, the investigators' institutions have been reluctant to defend their employees' right to publish, since they feared legal action. When such cases have come to light they have generated bad publicity for the companies involved. Two, well-publicised, cases are those of Nancy Olivieri[1] and Betty Dong.[2]

1 *Olivieri case*: Spurgeon D (2001) Report clears researcher who broke drug company agreement. *BMJ*. **323**: 1085.

2 *Dong case*: Rennie D (1998) Thyroid storm. *JAMA*. **277**: 1238–43.

Recognising the problems that can occur if there is no contract, GPP3 recommends written **publication agreements**.

If you are an academic researcher, you should check both your contract of employment with your institution, and any contracts you have for project funding. In particular, look out for any restrictions on publication, details about data ownership and requirements to review manuscripts before submission.

■ Contributorship (vs. authorship)

Some journals (in particular, the **'Big Five'**) recognise that authorship of research papers is a complex, even messy, business and have therefore shifted from a system of authorship to one of contributorship. This is also reflected in the latest version of the **International Committee of Medical Journal Editors' (ICJME)** guidelines. Instead of simply listing authors in the **by-line**, these journals provide an indication of each individual's contribution to the research and the publication. In recognition of the fact that each contributor may have had an input to only part of the project, these journals sometimes also require one contributor to act as **guarantor** for the project's overall integrity.

Authors/contributors therefore need to check the journal's requirements to see what information is required. If you plan to submit to a journal that lists contributors and their contributions, gather this information as soon as possible. Some journals provide a checklist, others leave it up to the contributors to write this section. In the latter case, it is particularly important that all co-authors (or should that be co-contributors?) agree the wording.

One reason why journals are switching to the contributorship system is to prevent **guest** or **ghost authors**. This should not be a problem if you have set up your **writing group** carefully and involved all the **key people/players**. Whether a journal uses a traditional author by-line or a contributor list, those listed should always meet agreed criteria for authorship.

The following references provide some background on the topic.

Horton R (1996) Signing up for authorship. *Lancet*. **347**: 780.

Rennie D (1997) When authorship fails. A proposal to make contributors accountable. *JAMA*. **278**: 579–85.

Smith R (1997) Authorship: time for a paradigm shift? *BMJ*. **314**: 992.

Wager E (2006) Bye-bye by line, hello contributors. *J R Soc Med*. **99**: 542–3.

■ COPE; *see* Committee on Publication Ethics

■ Copy editing; *see* technical editing

■ Copyright

If you want to reproduce a figure, a table or a large section of text from another publication you need permission from the copyright owner. Until recently, this was nearly always the journal or book publisher. Thus, authors needed permission to reproduce items from their own publications because they did not own the copyright. However, the situation has changed in recent years, and **Open Access journals** now allow authors to retain copyright in their own work.

Copyright relates to the way in which something appears on paper, i.e. the exact form of wording, or the precise form of a figure. It does not apply to the underlying data or ideas. Thus, if you present your data in another form, you will not be breaking copyright. Strictly speaking this means that if you redraw a graph and make some slight alterations to the labelling, you probably do not need permission. However, it is courteous to request permission, and this may prevent later problems. Large publishers have permissions departments which deal with such requests and usually handle them promptly. Some will ask for a fee (although this is rare for non-commercial uses), and most will stipulate the acknowledgement wording you should use.

Short quotations from other academic works do not require permission, but you should clearly indicate that these are quotations and cite the source. Publishers of song lyrics and modern fiction usually guard their copyright fiercely and may deny permission to quote, or charge a substantial fee, so make sure you get permission if you want to use a line from your favourite pop song as a catchy **title**.

Most journals require copies of permission letters on submission, so make your requests as soon as you decide to include copyright material in order to avoid delays later on.

■ Corporate integrity agreement (CIA)

Healthcare companies that have broken US marketing regulations may be subject to a CIA which aims to control their activities to make sure they don't do such naughty things again. The nature of the restrictions depends on the nature of the breach (or, as WS Gilbert put it, more succinctly, makes 'the punishment fit the crime'*). CIAs may affect the ways in which companies develop publication plans, for instance mandating author agreements, needs assessments and publication monitoring. A review of several CIAs concluded that they effectively enforced guidelines such as **Good Publication Practice** and the ICMJE Recommendations.[1] Anybody working in or for a company that has a CIA needs to be aware of any such requirements affecting publications.

1 Rodino FJ (2013) Corporate integrity statements: what they say about publications, publication planning, transparency, and ICMJE. *Ther Innov Regul Sci.* **41**: 50–6.

---

* In the same song, first performed in 1855, Gilbert even suggested a suitable punishment for false pharma advertising: 'The advertising quack who wearies with tales of countless cures, His teeth, I've enacted, shall all be extracted by terrified amateurs'.

■ Corrections (errata)

If, despite everybody's best care and attention, you discover an error in something you have published you should contact the journal and ask for a correction to be published. If the journal is indexed on Medline, corrections will be linked to the original article.

If you are feeling pedantic, you can impress the editor by knowing that the term 'correction' should be used for author errors and 'erratum' for the journal's own mistakes. If you want to be old-fashioned you can say 'corrigendum' instead of 'correction' (but they both mean that something has gone wrong).

■ Corresponding author

The corresponding author acts as the point of contact with the journal and will receive the reviewers' comments and proofs. The corresponding author's full contact details, or at least an e-mail address, are usually published with the paper so that readers can contact him/her and request reprints. For other authors, only the affiliation or a short address (e.g. hospital name and city) is usually published.

Since the corresponding author will receive reviewers' comments and proofs, it makes sense to choose the author who is least likely to move and who is most likely to be contactable and able to deal efficiently and rapidly with proofs.

While journals view the corresponding author as a purely administrative designation, some researchers and the UK Research Excellence Framework seem to equate this position with the study **guarantor**, or consider it indicates some degree of honour or prestige. It is hard to say whether readers share these views. *See* **order of authors** for more discussion on this tricky subject.

■ Council of Science Editors (CSE)

This was founded in 1957 as the Council of Biology Editors (CBE) and changed its name in 2000 to reflect its broader membership, although it still has a strong biomedical slant. Membership is open to anybody with an interest in science editing; professional North American journal editors and publishers are particularly well represented. CSE holds an annual meeting and occasional retreats, all in North America, and publishes *Science Editor*. The CSE website, www.councilscience editors.org, is an excellent resource containing thoughtful statements about a range of issues such as authorship. The meetings are a good way to meet editors, hear their concerns and maybe even buy them a beer.

■ Cover letter / covering letter

Do not overlook the task of composing a persuasive covering letter in the euphoria of having got everything agreed and the drudgery of sorting out the submission package. This is your chance to 'sell' your submission to the journal editor, but you should remain objective and avoid the 'hard sell'. Start by spelling the editor's name correctly and make sure you are addressing the current incumbent, not a long-deceased predecessor. Then describe your work in a few sentences and explain why you feel it is important. Make the editor's life easier and reap the benefits of careful journal selection by explaining how your work matches the journal's aims and scope, and will be of interest to its readers. If you are aiming at a particular section of the journal, or there is a choice of format (e.g. short or full reports) you should specify this. You should also show that you understand the journal's requirements, for instance by including a statement that the paper has not been published elsewhere and is not being considered by any other journals. Some journals stipulate the exact wording you must use for this and a few require only this standard text and give no opportunity for a traditional cover letter (see, for example, http://anesthesiology.pubs.asahq.org/SS/ASA_Cover_Letter.aspx). Many journals require authors to complete forms about **conflict of interest** but, if not, you should include a statement about this in your letter.

You will also need to write a covering letter when responding to reviewers' comments. Your response should always include a detailed list of the changes you have made and reasons why you have not followed a particular suggestion. This list may form part of your covering letter or may be a separate document.

■ Creative Commons (CC) licences

To fully comply with Open Access requirements (according to the 'Bethesda statement'[1]), publishers should use one of the variants of the CC licence. (Strictly speaking, if a journal makes its content freely available to readers but doesn't use such a licence, e.g. it demands copyright from the authors, it isn't Open Access, although this distinction is probably lost on many readers who are just happy they don't have to pay to read the articles.)

Full details are available at https://creativecommons.org/ (don't panic, although this site includes full legal wording for the licences for those who like that sort of thing, it also provides versions for normal people). Here's a quick summary.

Under a CC licence, the authors grant the publisher non-exclusive rights to publish their work while ensuring that they (i.e. the authors) retain the copyright. Unlike traditional copyright agreements, CC licences also allow other people to reuse or republish the work. The most permissive licence, CC-BY, allows anybody to reuse the work in any form so long as the source and authors are properly attributed. Other variants restrict reuse to non-commercial activities (CC-NC), restrict derivative works (ND) (essentially allowing only the original text version to be used rather than, say, a video or a translation), or restrict users to 'share alike' (SA) (i.e. they must use the same type of licence for any derivative works). These variants can be combined (e.g. CC-BY-NC).

A few publishers allow authors to select the type of CC licence that is used.

In this case, the choice is up to you. If you work for a commercial company, be aware that it might want to avoid an NC licence which would restrict its use of reprints. However, if you are an independent author you might prefer to prevent me (or a drug company or another publisher) from becoming rich by somehow reusing or reselling your precious work. Therefore, if authors have strong preferences, or a company has firm policies, about this, you should check what types of licence are offered by a particular journal. This information should be available (somewhere!) within the 'Instructions to authors', but can often be checked more quickly by looking at some recent articles which should display the CC logo and specify the type of licence (or indicate that a CC licence is not used, by displaying a traditional copyright marking).

1 Bethesda statement on open access publishing (2003). http://legacy.earlham.edu/~peters/fos/bethesda.htm

■ CrossCheck

Many journals screen text at some point for plagiarism, and the majority use a system called CrossCheck, which is provided by CrossRef (the not-for-profit collaboration that provides **DOI**s). This system combines text-matching software from a company called iParadigms (which produces Turnitin, which is widely used to check for plagiarism in academia) with a huge database of books and journals supplied by publishers. This enables the software to look for matches within journals that are behind access barriers, which would not show up on a regular Google search.

Publication planners and honest authors (who have no intention of committing plagiarism) need to know about CrossCheck because it is also highly sensitive to **redundant publication** (sometimes known as 'text recycling'). If you are writing several reports from a single study or dataset, or even a series of trials on the same treatment or therapy area, it may be tempting to copy and paste sections from previous introduction or discussion sections. Most journal editors understand that such recycling may be unavoidable, as there may be only a few ways to state something clearly (for example, a fact such as 'one in twelve women will develop breast cancer'). But bear in mind that text-matching software isn't able to think, and usually picks up any string of six or more words, so such innocent repetition could lead to questions from the journal. Writers therefore need to be cautious when reusing their own words and ultra-scrupulous to avoid lifting words from other people's publications without using quotation marks or paraphrasing (as well as clearly referencing the source). If you are worried that a journal might accuse you of **text recycling** (e.g. in a secondary publication) you could demonstrate your honesty by mentioning any overlapping publications in your covering letter. Editors are generally so accustomed to, and annoyed by, authors failing to mention related publications and trying to get away with salami slicing that they are likely to be impressed by this.

■ CrossMark

This is a really neat innovation provided by CrossRef (the not-for-profit collaboration that provides DOIs and CrossCheck). It creates a permanent link to the so-called 'publisher-curated version' of an article – in other words, the most up-to-date one. Even if somebody has downloaded a PDF onto their computer, if they click this link they can see if the article has been corrected or retracted. Use of CrossMarks, while unlikely to be the deciding factor when selecting your target journal, is a sign that the publisher has invested in this helpful technology and takes their responsibilities to readers seriously.

www.crossref.org/crossmark/

■ CSE; *see* Council of Science Editors

D

■ Data access; *see* access to data

■ Data analysis plan

Statistical analysis is a crucial part of research methodology. Every trial plan, no matter how straightforward, should therefore include a description of how the data will be analysed. This may form part of the trial protocol or a separate data (or statistical) analysis plan (SAP). Somebody with statistical expertise should advise on the appropriate methods to use. The plan should set out the primary endpoints of the study and will often include a power calculation to indicate the sample size needed to confirm or refute the underlying hypothesis with confidence. Whatever the **key message(s)** of the publication, it is important to distinguish primary outcomes from secondary or post hoc analyses. The data analysis plan should help to ensure that a study is analysed and reported responsibly. A medical writer preparing a draft should have access to the plan to determine the primary endpoints and for details such as power calculations and randomisation methods which are required to fulfil the **CONSORT** requirements. Some journals (e.g. *JAMA*) require a copy of the statistical analysis plan to accompany submissions of manuscripts reporting clinical trials.

Developing the initial publication strategy and the data analysis plan at the same time can save a lot of time and trouble later. For example, if you consider what tables you might include in a publication you can ensure that the analysis will provide these.

■ Data dredging

This disparaging term refers to the practice of analysing data well beyond any reasonable scientific or statistical bounds in a desperate search for significant-looking p-values or the hope of wringing out some publication-worthy droplets. It therefore tends to result in **redundant publications**, or even to completely fallacious ones. The simple rule to avoid data dredging is to have a **data analysis plan** and stick to it. Occasionally, post hoc analyses will be justified if you notice interesting patterns in your data or want to explore a new hypothesis, but always seek the advice of a statistician about the validity of such analyses and, if you do try to publish them, make sure secondary analyses are clearly labelled as such and that appropriate statistical methods have been used to correct for multiple analyses.

■ Data ownership; *see* ownership of data

■ DataVision

Web-based publication planning software developed by Envision Pharma. It provides project management tools and databases giving information about journals and congresses. See www.envisionpharma.com for details.

■ Deadlines

Meetings usually have strict deadlines for **abstract** submission. Occasionally, exceptions can be made and abstracts accepted after the deadline, but do not count on this. Generally, the larger the meeting, the firmer the deadline. If you know your results will only be available a few days after the deadline it might be worth contacting the meeting organisers and asking if they can extend the deadline or if **late breaker abstracts** will be accepted. Try to do this as far in advance as possible. Submission deadlines sometimes get extended if the organisers receive fewer abstracts than they had hoped for – but, again, you should not count on this, even if it has happened in previous years.

The only deadline you are likely to encounter from a journal is one for returning proofs. After waiting several months for these to arrive, this can sometimes be unexpectedly short, e.g. 48 hours. Failure to return corrected proofs within this deadline may delay publication until the next issue. This is why it makes sense to inform the journal if the **corresponding author**'s contact details change, and to nominate somebody for this role who is likely to respond quickly.

■ Decision times

Although electronic submission and reviewing may have trimmed a few days off journal schedules, external reviewers remain the rate-limiting step in the peer-review process. Most journals do not pay their reviewers (or offer only a nominal reward) so editors cannot demand a rapid response. Good reviewers are also hard to find, so editors are keen not to antagonise or overburden them. Because of this, authors often have to wait several weeks, and sometimes several months, for a decision from traditional journals. (The median time from submission to acceptance for *JAMA* in 2014 was 35 days but that represents a considerable improvement from the 103-day average in 2004.) However, in journals that use in-house review to screen all submissions, average times for rejection may be much shorter than those for acceptance. (The median time from receipt to rejection at *JAMA* in 2014 was just 4 days.)

Aware of the frustration caused by waiting for decisions, and also of the fact that drug companies may be prepared to pay for a more rapid service, some journals offer rapid review for a fee. For example, the *International Journal of Clinical Practice* offers an expedited review service that ensures peer review within 7 days of online submission and proofs within 7 days of acceptance. However, expedited review is only available for clinical trials (which must conform with the **CONSORT** or STROBE reporting guidelines). *Current Medical Research & Opinion* offers RapidTrack peer review within 4 weeks and submission to online publication in 8–10 weeks or FastTrack peer review within 2 weeks with submission to online publication in 4–6 weeks.

Do not confuse journals that offer quick decisions for all or some papers with the practice of having a **fast-track publication** route for papers of exceptional interest. Remember that the editor will decide whether your paper merits special treatment and, by definition, this is only going to apply to a few, remarkable studies. If speed of publication is important, it is better to select your target journal carefully than to rely on rapid review in a big-name journal.

See also **acceptance times** and **rejection** times and Chapter 3 'How long will it take?' (pp. 13–17) for more details.

■ DeepDyve

Authors should not cite references they have not read (e.g. by copying information from another publication, including the citation). However, unless you have access to a good institutional library, it can be difficult or expensive to obtain all the references you might need to prepare your article. One way of reading articles but avoiding the high costs of 'pay-per-view' charges is to use DeepDyve (available at www.deepdyve.com).

This facility allows you to access and read (but *not* save a copy of) articles from certain publishers that would otherwise be behind a pay wall. This could be useful if you need to check a fact cited in another publication. (Several studies have shown that misquotation is a worryingly common problem so it really does make sense to check the original source and not rely on other authors' interpretations.) If you are being conscientious, you should obtain a full copy of all articles you actually cite, but if you take careful notes, then reading something via DeepDyve is definitely better than citing something if you have only read the abstract, or if you haven't read it at all, and may be helpful if you need to screen many articles (e.g. after doing a literature search) but want to avoid paying for those that aren't relevant.

■ Diamond Open Access

This term is used to describe Open Access journals that do not charge authors an **article processing charge**. Such generosity is usually made possible by subsidies from academic societies or foundations. It is sometimes also called 'Platinum Open Access'. This is a useful option if you are keen to publish in an Open Access journal but can't afford the fees; however, its usefulness is limited by the fact that very few medical journals run this way.

Fuchs C and Sandoval M (2013) The diamond model of open access publishing: why policy makers, scholars, universities, libraries, labour unions and the publishing world need to take non-commercial, non-profit open access serious. *Triple C*. **11**: 428–43.

Taylor & Francis (2013) Open access. http://editorresources.taylorandfrancisgroup.com/open-access/

■ Directory of Open Access Journals (DOAJ)

This directory lists over 10 000 Open Access journals covering a range of disciplines. DOAJ members are expected to follow the 'Principles of transparency and best practice in scholarly publishing'[1] set out in 2014 in response to concerns about predatory Open Access publishers (*see* **predatory publishers**). It is a useful resource if you are searching for Open Access journals; however, membership of DOAJ is not necessarily a guarantee of high standards, as revealed when a journalist submitted fake articles to journals from the list and found that many accepted the articles with only cursory review, despite serious flaws.[2]

1 DOAJ (2014) Principles of transparency and best practice in scholarly publishing. https://doaj.org/bestpractice

2 Bohannon J (2013) Who's afraid of peer review? *Science*. **342**: 60–5.

■ DOI (Digital Object Identifier) system

The DOI system was introduced to overcome some of the difficulties of citing electronic material. It is administered by the International DOI Foundation, which defines a DOI as 'a persistent identifier of intellectual property entities'. Some journals now assign a DOI to every article. They act like a postcode and could, in theory, replace traditional citations, but since they are long, unmemorable strings of numbers and letters, this seems unlikely unless human intelligence evolves unexpectedly. DOIs are especially useful for citing electronic references, **supplementary material** or items posted on a journal's website before the print edition which have not yet had volume or page numbers assigned. The system also forms the basis for CrossRef, a not-for-profit initiative that allows publishers to cross-link citations so readers can go directly from an article to a cited reference in a few mouse clicks.

For more information go to www.doi.org or www.crossref.org.

■ Duplicate publication; *see* redundant publication

E

■ EASE; *see* European Association of Science Editors

■ Economic (health outcomes) evaluations

These are often published as secondary papers (i.e. separately from the original clinical trial results) in specialist health economics journals. However, such journals tend to be read by economists rather than by prescribers. Some editors consider that economic aspects can only be evaluated in the context of clinical findings and, for this reason, *The BMJ* will not accept economic evaluations without the clinical results.[1] Introduced in 2002, this policy does not seem to have been adopted by other journals or incorporated in the **International Committee of Medical Journal Editors' (ICMJE)** 'Recommendations for the conduct, reporting, editing, and publication of scholarly work in medical journals', but it is worth checking instructions carefully in case your target journal has a similar policy. For guidelines on reporting health economics *see* the **Consolidated Health Economic Evaluation Reporting Standards (CHEERS)**.

1 Smith R (2002) New BMJ policy on economic evaluations. *BMJ*. **325**: 1124.

■ Editorial board

Most journals have editorial boards but their composition and role vary greatly. Having a contact on the editorial board might be an advantage, but in order to appreciate just how much (or how little) influence this person may have, you need to understand the board's role in a particular journal. Editorial board members are usually listed on the journal website or inside the front cover. The first thing to do is count them. If your chum is one of dozens, then his or her influence is likely to be limited. If, on the other hand, there are fewer than 12 members, you might really have a friend at court. Next look at the journal's 'Instructions to contributors'. If members of the editorial board are assigned to handle certain papers, this suggests they may perform an important screening function and may act, in effect, as the editor for their region or subject area. Finally, try to find out if and when the editorial board meets. The strongest clue to this is given in journals that publish acceptance dates for papers: if the papers published in each issue seem to have been accepted on only one or two dates, this suggests an active editorial board that meets to decide what to accept. In contrast, some journals use their editorial board mainly as a figurehead in which case it will meet only rarely (if at all) and its members are virtually never used as reviewers – let alone expected to discuss the fate of papers. In this case, it may do no harm to contact your friend to ask his or her general advice about whether your paper is suited to the journal, but you cannot expect much more. In the worst case, board members may be dead (making them especially hard to contact and unlikely to intercede on your behalf).

See **review process** for more details about how journals organise their peer review.

■ Editorials

In many journals, editorials or commentaries accompany research papers or comment on important developments. Such 'opinion pieces' are usually commissioned by the journal, often from somebody who reviewed the paper or who is an expert in the field. In *The Lancet*, the editorials are always written by a member of staff and appear under the **by-line** 'Lancet'. However, the journal also publishes commentaries. If you have an idea for an editorial or commentary it is best to contact the editor informally to discover whether the journal considers uncommissioned pieces, and, if so, whether it might be interested in yours. Editorials to accompany an article may have to be prepared quickly so as not to delay publication.

The purpose of editorials and commentaries is to present the commentator's views on the meaning of a publication or the implications of a new policy or development. They usually contain a few references but can include more unsubstantiated opinion than other types of publication.

Since they express an opinion, it is important that the writer's voice is heard, and it is usually inappropriate for another party to suggest what the author should write or how they should tackle the subject. For this reason, the first version of the

Good Publication Practice (GPP) guidelines for pharmaceutical companies recommended that, while it is acceptable for a professional writer or editor to polish an editorial for an author (e.g. to help a non-native English speaker), it is not usually acceptable for anybody other than the named author to prepare the first draft.

■ Editors

There are several types of editor and it is important to understand their different roles. The Editor (or Editor-in-Chief) of a journal is the overall boss, having the final decision over what gets published and responsibility for setting the journal's policies. He or she may be advised and assisted by committees, editorial boards and junior editors, but, the Editor (with a capital 'E') carries final responsibility. Editors may be full-time professionals employed by the journal (or its parent organisation) or part-timers doing their editing job on top of another. Full-time Editors usually work from a journal or publisher's office, while part-time ones usually work from their own institution. The level of administrative support available to different types of editors therefore varies. If you contact a secretary or assistant in a journal office it is reasonable to expect that s/he is familiar with the journal's processes and may have access to files. On the other hand, a secretary in a university or hospital may have virtually nothing to do with her boss' editorial responsibilities.

Working alongside the Editor may be assistant editors with responsibility for sections of the journal (e.g. correspondence) or a proportion of submissions. Finally, there is another species of editor responsible for preparing accepted typescripts for printing. These are called technical editors, desk editors or sub-editors depending on the journal. This type of editor takes no part in deciding what gets published but will put submissions into **house style** and check proofs (*see* **technical editing** for more details). If you find major problems in the proofs, it is usually best to discuss them directly with the sub-editor who prepared the manuscript. In the case of journals edited by part-time editors, technical editing may be done by somebody employed (or hired) by the academic society or publisher, or by the Editor. Check the contact details supplied with the proofs to determine the best person to contact.

To complete the classification, we should not forget authors' editors who help authors prepare submissions. They may be employed by the authors' institution (especially in the case of large US universities) or may be freelance.

■ Electronic publishing

Many journals that started life, and are still firmly rooted, in traditional paper and print use the internet or electronic media to some extent. They have been joined by wholly electronic publications that exist solely on the internet. The term 'electronic publishing' seems to cover all aspects of this wide spectrum, making it, unless clearly defined, rather meaningless.

However, when choosing a journal you should consider how it is published, since this will affect not only the speed of publication but also the journal's accessibility and how it is likely to be perceived. Medical journals fall into two broad categories – those that are purely electronic, such as the **BioMed Central** and **Public Library of Science (PLOS)** journals, and those that still use print as the version of record but offer various electronic functions, such as *The Lancet*. A few, such as *The BMJ*, are true hybrids, offering longer versions of papers and extra features such as rapid responses on the website. If you have very large data tables, or want to include media such as video clips, it is worth considering journals that can publish **supplementary material** electronically.

Since purely electronic journals are not constrained by production and distribution costs (and therefore do not have to work within a page budget) they often have higher acceptance rates than print journals. Electronic journals also tend to have a considerably shorter **lead time** from acceptance to publication since articles do not have to wait for the next printed issue. On the negative side, electronic journals tend to invest less in **technical editing** than printed ones, and, being newer and easier to get into are generally considered less prestigious. As well as traditional journal metrics, some electronic journals now offer article-level metrics so you can see how many people have downloaded or cited your work (the PLOS system is explained at http://article-level-metrics.plos.org). Some journals also encourage readers to rate, annotate or comment on articles, which could be great if they say nice things about your research but not so welcome if they are critical.

Other benefits are that most electronic publications are **Open Access journals**, or are available via **PubMed Central**, reducing the importance of indexing.

Although not strictly related to their electronic status, some of the newer journals practise open (unblinded) peer review, and some (such as *BMJ Open* and many of those published by **BioMed Central**) take this one stage further by making reviewers' comments available to readers.

■ Electronic review

Most journals use e-mail to communicate with reviewers. Although this has several advantages, and should, in theory, shorten review time, it probably has not accelerated the process enormously, as the rate-limiting step remains the busy (and unpaid) reviewer. On a less curmudgeonly note, electronic review does offer potential advantages, such as automatic links to references cited in the submission, or to guidelines for reviewers. It also enables potential reviewers to read an **abstract** before deciding whether to accept the invitation to review – this might help to identify competing interests earlier, although a study at *Annals of Emergency Medicine* suggested that it does not speed up the review process.

■ Electronic submission

Nearly all journals permit or even mandate electronic submission of articles via their website. Check the 'Instructions to contributors' for details of file formats, etc. that are acceptable. Formatting details that often cause problems (and which journals therefore often ask you to remove) include fixed page breaks, right-hand justification and tables aligned using spaces rather than tabs or table settings. Special characters such as Greek letters or accents often get lost in transmission. It is therefore safer to use alternatives such as mcg for micrograms (rather than µg) or spelling out alpha and beta. Pay careful attention to special characters when you paste text into a form for submitting an abstract to a conference – I have seen very odd things happen to Greek characters and symbols, such as less than (<).

Even if you submit a paper or abstract electronically, you may still have to send hard copies of signed forms such as copyright transfers or authorship statements.

Many conferences now send automatic acknowledgements of electronically submitted abstracts, which is reassuring. However, as with any submission, you should make a note when you do it and contact the journal or meeting if you have received no acknowledgement after about a month. Both paper and electronic submissions do sometimes get lost in transmission, or at the editorial office, so it is reasonable to expect some sort of acknowledgement.

■ ELPS

This acronym is used by *The BMJ* to stand for Electronic Long, Paper Short[1] referring to the fact that articles in the printed version are shorter than those on the website. Although most journals do not go as far as *The BMJ* (which invests heavily in editors who trim the paper version) many with websites will post **supplementary material**, such as large data tables, copies of questionnaires or video clips, which cannot be accommodated in the printed version.

If you have a lot of data to present, or want to use an unconventional medium (such as video), study the journal's website, check the 'Instructions to authors' or contact the editorial office to see if they can handle this.

1 See Müllner M and Groves T (2002) Making research papers in the *BMJ* more accessible. *BMJ*. **325**: 456 and Schroter S, Barratt H and Smith J (2004) Authors' perceptions of electronic publishing: two cross-sectional surveys. *BMJ*. **328**: 1350–3.

■ Embargoes

Journals often issue press releases a little before the publication date but with an embargo to prevent journalists publishing anything before this date. The idea is to give journalists time to research and write their story but to prevent press coverage before the full article is available. Journals also expect authors not to release details about forthcoming publications. For example, *JAMA* states 'All information regarding the content and publication date of accepted manuscripts is strictly confidential. Unauthorized prepublication release of accepted manuscripts and information about planned publication date may result in rescinding the acceptance and rejecting the paper'. *See also* **Media relations**.

■ Encore abstracts

This term may be used to describe similar or identical abstracts, describing the same results, submitted to more than one conference. While cries of 'Encore!' at the opera house are regarded as a sign of success, similar cries at academic meetings may be less welcome. Although some meetings will accept abstracts describing results that have already been presented elsewhere, and such abstracts are not usually considered as redundant publication, some people have criticised the practice and some company policies discourage or prohibit it.

While it may not be unethical to send the same abstract to several meetings, there are some practical considerations. First, you should check that the meeting allows this. Some large meetings will only consider new findings, but smaller, local meetings are often happy to accept encore presentations. Second, you should check who holds the copyright on the abstract (although, to be honest, many people ignore this). If the abstract is published in a journal or website then copyright may have been transferred to the publisher or conference organiser, in which case you would need permission to republish it. Remember, too, that most conferences will not consider work that has already been published in full, and a long series of repeats might delay full publication in a journal. The major pharmaceutical industry organisations (PhRMA, EFPIA, JPMA) recommend that results should be published 'no later than 18 months after study end' and some companies set more ambitious targets.

GPP3 is one of the few guidelines to cover conference presentations as well as journal publications. It states 'A repeat presentation of the data to different congresses is permissible to reach different audiences, provided the congress permits this "encore" presentation and copyright requirements are respected. Encore presentations should usually have the same authorship as the original presentation. However, authorship of encore presentations at national or local meetings may differ slightly (e.g., to enable presentation in the appropriate language in situations where the congress does not allow nonauthor presenters), provided all original authors agree.'

■ Enhanced publications

Many journals now offer additional publication options that go beyond the traditional words and diagrams of a classic article, such as videos, podcasts, animations and slide sets. If these are important to you, you should include them in your criteria for choosing a target journal as the possibilities do vary between publishers. If you are working for a company, you may also need to check how any such supplementary materials will be reviewed or approved as they may fall into the category of marketing material which is usually regulated and therefore handled differently from articles in peer-reviewed journals. For example, if a company pays for an author to make a short video describing a study about their product, and this is then posted on a journal website, this might be regarded as a form of advertising (whereas the article it related to would not).

Here are some examples of journals' multimedia offerings:

- *The BMJ* videos: www.youtube.com/user/BMJmedia
- *JAMA* author interviews: http://jama.jamanetwork.com/multimedia.aspx#AuthorInterviews
- *The Lancet* podcasts: www.thelancet.com/audio
- *The New England Journal of Medicine* interactive medical cases: www.nejm.org/multimedia/interactive-medical-case
- *Annals of Internal Medicine* cartoons: http://annals.org/SS/graphicmedicine.aspx
- Elsevier audio slides: www.elsevier.com/books-and-journals/content-innovation/audioslides

See also **supplementary material**.

■ Envision

Commercial company that provides **DataVision** publication planning tools which are used by many companies.

■ e-Prints; *see preprints*

■ epub

This term is used on **Medline** (usually as 'epub ahead of print') to indicate an article that has been published electronically but has not yet appeared in the printed version of the journal. Such articles are considered fully published (i.e. they are no longer 'in press') but they may not yet have journal volume or page numbers assigned. However, they can be cited using their **DOI**.

■ EQUATOR Network

An international initiative to improve the reporting of medical research. It was started by members of the team that developed **CONSORT** but their resource centre gives useful links to a wide range of guidelines (almost 300 at the last count) so this website is a good place to check if there are any guidelines on the type of research you are trying to publish.

www.equator-network.org

■ Errata; *see corrections*

■ European Association of Science Editors (EASE)

This was founded in 1982 from the merger of the European Life Sciences Editors Association and Editerra, an association for earth science editors. Membership is not restricted to Europe, and EASE currently has members from over 50 countries.

EASE holds meetings every two or three years. Unlike **WAME** and **CSE**, EASE has not issued statements on editorial policy, but it has produced a handbook for editors. It publishes *European Science Editing* which includes peer-reviewed research articles as well as association news and useful summaries of papers about all aspects of editing and publishing. Membership of EASE includes academic (i.e. part-time) editors, technical editors and translators, as well as professional editors and publishers.

For more information look at www.ease.org.uk.

■ European Clinical Trials Database (EudraCT)

This trial register contains information about all trials reported to the European regulatory authorities since 2004. However, EudraCT has only been opened to the public (and therefore recognised as meeting the ICMJE requirements for trial registration) since June 2011. Europe has been slower than the USA in requiring trial sponsors to post summary results of clinical trials on its database. Whereas this has been required for new products in the USA since 2008, it only came into force in Europe in July 2014, although results of studies in children have been available since 2007, as these were governed by a separate directive. Fortunately (for publication planners) both the US and EU authorities have set similar deadlines for posting results summaries: for most trials these must be posted within 12 months of the study end. Posting such a summary does not constitute prior publication and therefore does not prevent trials being published in journals but the timing may affect publication strategies since sponsors may aim to ensure that a full description is available in a journal by the time the summary appears on EudraCT and **ClinicalTrials.gov**.

https://eudract.ema.europa.eu/index.html

www.clinicaltrialsregister.eu/about.html

■ European Federation of Pharmaceutical Industry Associations (EFPIA)

An umbrella group of national industry organisations in Europe (such as the Association of the British Pharmaceutical Industry), EFPIA occasionally produces statements (often in conjunction with the US industry body, PhRMA) relating to publication. One of the most relevant is the statement on the publication of clinical trial results issued in 2010.[1] This recommends that all industry-sponsored trials should be 'considered for publication' regardless of whether findings are positive or negative, and that clinical trial results should be submitted for publication no later than 18 months after the end of the study.

1 www.efpia.eu/uploads/Modules/Documents/20100610_joint_position_publication_10jun2010.pdf

■ European Medical Writers Association (EMWA)

As the name suggests, this is an organisation for medical writers in Europe. It developed from the American Medical Writers Association (AMWA) in 1989 and now largely functions independently. EMWA has produced guidelines on the role of professional medical writers in developing publications (available at www.emwa.org/documents/about_us/EMWAguidelines.pdf).

For more details visit www.emwa.org.

Jacobs A and Wager E (2005) European Medical Writers Association (EMWA) guidelines on the role of medical writers in developing peer-reviewed publications. *Curr Med Res Opin*. **21**: 317–21.

■ Expectations

A publication is usually the end-product of a collaboration involving many people. Devising, agreeing and communicating a successful publication strategy therefore depends on discovering the expectations of everybody involved. Depending on their background, previous experience and personality, people can have widely different expectations. Do not assume that you know what individuals hope to get out of a publication, or what they expect the processes will be.

The relationship between research sponsors and investigators can be a complex and delicate one. Involvement of extra parties such as contract research organisations (CROs), communications agencies or freelance professional writers can add further layers of complexity. The first step in establishing expectations is to make sure that all **key players** have been consulted and offered the chance to contribute. For large studies, this is likely to involve a wider group than just the named authors.

The best way to find out what people expect is to arrange a **meeting** involving as many key players as possible. If this is difficult, a telephone or video conference is probably the next best thing. Appoint somebody to chair the meeting or lead the phone conference, and somebody else to record the decisions.

When discussing a publication strategy try to cover all the issues. The most important ones to establish are:

- timing
- target meetings (for abstracts)
- target journal (for primary publication)
- number of publications
- authorship
- key messages
- roles (i.e. who does what).

When these are agreed, write them down and circulate the information. Memories are unreliable, and written notes will also help to inform those who could not take part in the discussion.

If circumstances change, keep checking expectations and consulting the key players. Always consider if you have left anybody out (e.g. an investigator who might expect to be an author). If in doubt, increase your communication network rather than narrowing it. Differences in expectations are best settled well before crucial deadlines (e.g. for abstract submission) and at the earliest stages of publication development.

The best way of checking expectations on a full paper is to circulate an **outline** for comment before preparing a first draft. It is far better to uncover differences in interpretation and emphasis at this stage than when you are just about to submit the paper.

Many publishing conventions are unwritten. I have been mystified by authors squabbling over who should be named as the **corresponding author**, or why they like the convention that male authors are listed with their initials, but female authors have their forenames spelled out in full. Even experienced researchers can have strange misconceptions about publication processes, and everybody has their own idiosyncrasies, prejudices and opinions. The only method to guarantee a smooth process is to make no assumptions, discover everybody's expectations about what should happen and keep the lines of communication open.

■ Expedited review

A posh term for a fast-track review system which some journals offer for a fee. *See* **decision times** for more details.

■ External review

The traditional model of peer review, and probably the one that most authors expect journals to use, involves sending papers to external reviewers (i.e. independent experts who are not employed by the journal). However, journals that employ a large editorial team reject a considerable proportion of submissions without external review. Such journals (which tend to be the large, general weekly journals such as *The Lancet* and *NEJM*) always use external reviewers before papers are accepted, but they reject as many as 30–50% of submissions on internal review. The advantage of internal screening (or **in-house review**) is that it usually produces a rapid decision. The disadvantage is that authors receive a less detailed critique – often just a letter stating that the submission is not suitable for the journal.

F

■ *F1000Research*

This journal has several unusual features which, depending on your point of view, may increase or decrease its attractiveness as a target for your work. First, it will only publish work for which the raw data is made publicly available. Second, it posts submissions on a public website before inviting reviewers to appraise them. This offers the advantage of speed (your work is accessible immediately) but the disadvantage that if the reviews are unfavourable you almost certainly cannot submit your work to another journal. The third slightly unusual (but by no means unique) feature is that reviewer comments are published alongside the article.

The post-publication peer review model raises interesting philosophical questions about what exactly publication is and also serious practical questions about what happens to articles that do not receive favourable reviews and are therefore not accepted for publication. Leaving aside the fascinating but tough question of what we mean by publication, the answer to the easier, second question is that *F1000Research* encourages authors to continue to revise their manuscript until the reviewers are happy with it – even if this involves doing extra experiments or reanalysing the data. However, if, after endless revisions, the reviewers still do not give a favourable opinion, the article remains accessible to those who know it's there (since it has an electronic reference, or **DOI [digital object identifier]**) but it is not entered onto the journal's index or sent for indexing in other systems such as **PubMed Central** so it won't be picked up in literature searches.

See also **preprints** for more variants on the peer-review process.

■ Fast-track publication

Some journals offer rapid publication (within about 4 weeks of acceptance) for papers that represent major breakthroughs or have important public health implications. However, apart from a few journals that offer ultra-speedy publication if you pay an extra fee, you cannot generally demand a place on the fast-track just because it is convenient for you. The decision to accept a paper as fast-track rests with the editor. Few papers are deemed worthy of fast-tracking, so you will need to construct a very persuasive **covering letter** to explain exactly why your paper merits special attention. *The Lancet*'s instructions to contributors recommend calling the editor for a preliminary discussion. Since only a handful of exceptional papers will be afforded this honour, you should not expect fast-track as a right. After you have devoted years of your life to a piece of research you are bound to believe it is of enormous importance. Try to take a step back or get your most sceptical colleagues' views before assuming that your paper will qualify. Very few individual studies answer an important question so clearly that they change the practice of medicine. Mostly, science evolves gradually and your research will represent one piece of a larger jigsaw. If speed of publication is vital, it is better to choose your target journal carefully than to rely on fast-track review in a major journal. Some journals that cater mainly to pharmaceutical industry needs routinely offer rapid decisions and minimal **lead time** from acceptance to publication, and, as these journals generally also have higher acceptance rates than traditional, highly selective print journals, this is undoubtedly a more reliable route to guarantee prompt publication.

The conference equivalent of the journal's fast-track is **late breaker abstracts**.

Goldbeck-Wood S (1999) *BMJ* introduces a fast track system for papers. *BMJ*. **318**: 620, but see also an alternative view: Martyn C (2005) Slow tracking for *BMJ* papers. *BMJ*. **331**: 1551–2.

■ FDAAA

This rather unpronounceable acronym stands for the equally unwieldy Food and Drug Administration Amendments Act of 2007. The Act requires tabular summaries of the results of most Phase II to IV studies to be posted on **ClinicalTrials.gov** within 12 months of the study ending. In response to this, some drug companies now try to publish a full paper in a journal by about the same time as the results summary is posted, to provide context and interpretation to complement the very dry summary tables. This can set tough deadlines for publication planners who therefore do not have time to say 'FDA Amendments Act' and refer to it as 'Fe-daah'.

Wager E (2008) *FDAAA Legislation: Global Implications for Clinical Trial Reporting and Publication Planning*. Keyword Pharma Report 2008. www.keywordpharma.com/prods/wager3.asp

■ Fees; *see* article processing charge (APC)

■ Figure legends

Requirements for these may vary but many journals expect figure legends (headings) to be listed all together at the end of the document rather than with each figure. This reflects the old printing technology in which words were typeset along with the text while figures had to be processed and inserted separately and newer technology that requires figures to be prepared with graphics software rather than Word. Even if your software allows you to insert figures into a document, many journals require you to submit them as separate files, with the legends listed after the text.

Aim to make figure legends comprehensible to someone who has only scanned the text, for example by spelling out abbreviations. References in legends can cause problems, especially if the journal uses the Vancouver (sequential numbering) system, since you cannot tell exactly where the figure will appear in the text until the pages are made up. It is therefore helpful to refer to the author and date, as well as giving a number. If a figure is taken from another work you must obtain **permission** from the copyright holder (*see* **copyright**) and it is usual to mention this in the legend. If a figure has been adapted from another source it is courteous to acknowledge this even though you may not require formal permission. Typical wording would be:

> Fig. X. The renin-angiotensin system (reproduced from Baggins *et al.*[Ref c] by permission of Journals-R-Us Inc.).

■ Figures

The familiar equation that 'a picture is worth a thousand words' does not necessarily hold in scientific publishing. The 'rules' governing figures are often unwritten, and are definitely different for posters and papers.

Posters at conferences tend to be skimmed rapidly, rather than read, so the aim is to get your message across quickly and clearly. Figures such as flow diagrams, bar charts and pie charts are effective ways to display study designs and results, and should be used freely. If space permits, you can even show data both in a table and a graph (a luxury not permitted in a paper). Use your judgement to choose between including a lot of detail, and presenting clean, clear graphics. Some details, such as error bars, may be essential for understanding the data, others, such as exact patient numbers for every parameter measured, may be unnecessary. Pie charts and stacked bars are good for showing differences in proportions. Bar charts are good for comparing pairs of data, such as mean values from different treatment groups. Line graphs are good for showing changes over time. Use colours consistently (e.g. to indicate different treatment groups) and avoid red/

green contrasts since about one in 12 men have some degree of colour-blindness and cannot distinguish these colours.

Journals often impose restrictions on the number and type of figures you can include in a paper. The general rule is that you must not duplicate information between text, tables and figures. You must therefore choose the best form for presenting your data. Unlike posters, papers are usually considered the 'publication of record', in other words, the definitive and lasting report of a piece of research. Papers may be used for systematic reviews or meta-analyses which require considerable detail. For these reasons (and, perhaps because, in the past, typesetting and reproducing figures cost more than printing text or tables) journal editors usually favour tables over figures.

A simple bar chart comparing values from two groups is unlikely to be accepted in a paper. It is usually best to present this sort of data in a table, which allows you to show the actual values, a measure of the dispersion (e.g. standard deviation) and a measure of the effect size or statistical significance (e.g. 95% confidence interval or p-value).

However, other kinds of figures, such as those that synthesise a lot of data points, are usually acceptable, for example scatter plots or regression analyses and survival curves (e.g. Kaplan-Meier plots). Line graphs showing changes over several time points can also be useful if they complement the text or table rather than duplicate it.

Images such as X-rays, CT-scans or photomicrographs can be useful in case reports or to illustrate an unusual finding within a study. Photographs of patients may also be useful, but should be included only if you have obtained specific consent from the subject. It is not acceptable simply to blank out the eyes in an attempt to anonymise an image. Some journals require evidence of patient consent for publication. Make sure that images such as CT- and ultrasound scans do not contain details that might identify the subject.

If you want to reproduce a figure from another publication (even one of your own) you must obtain permission from the **copyright** owner (usually the publisher, but *see* the section on **permissions** for details). Many journals require evidence that permission has been obtained, so sort this out in good time before you plan to submit.

When preparing a paper, figures are usually presented separately, at the end of a document or in separate files. Even though your word processor will allow you to embed figures in the text, you should not do so (unless, of course, the journal requires this). Some journals also require figure legends to be submitted separately from the figures. (This convention dates back to old printing technology in which text was typeset separately and figures were then slotted into the pages. Although this is now obsolete, some journals still request it, and obeying their request shows that you have, at least, read their instructions which will, no doubt, please the old-fashioned editors who still require it.)

Most journals do not use colour printing for papers, and those that do (e.g. *The Lancet* has gone technicolour) will convert your figures into their colour scheme.

Graphics should therefore be prepared in black and white. Some journals charge to include colour photographs – check the instructions for details.

Many software packages such as Excel and Lotus allow you to prepare simple figures. However, if you want to add error bars or use more sophisticated graphics you will need specialist software. Remember that figures are usually produced larger than they will appear in print, so labels, in particular, must survive reduction. The default settings for label size on programs such as Excel or PowerPoint are designed for printing on A4 (or 8" × 11") paper or preparing slides, so they are usually too small. Before spending a lot of time preparing your own graphs, check the formats acceptable to the journal. (BioMed Central lists some programs that may enable you to convert files into a format suitable for publication at www.biomedcentral.com/authors/authortools.) It may save a lot of time to get graphs drawn by a professional illustrator who can supply formats such as .eps files which can be submitted electronically to journals, or high quality glossy prints suitable for printing.

If you are planning a budget for getting a paper published, remember to include the cost of preparing figures and for copyright charges (if you want to reproduce published figures). It may often be quicker and cheaper, and the results certainly more appealing, to get figures professionally drawn than to expect investigators or writers to produce them.

Many journals have specific guidelines for preparing digital images to prevent fraudulent manipulation. If an image has been cropped or edited, some journals will also require the original (i.e. uncropped) to check that the editing is acceptable. *The Journal of Cell Biology* (*JCB*) was one of the first to highlight the problem of image manipulation and has produced detailed guidelines which have been adopted by other journals.

JCB guidelines on figure preparation: http://jcb.rupress.org/site/misc/print.xhtml#digim

Rossner M and Yamada KM (2004). What's in a picture? The temptation of image manipulation. *J Cell Biol.* **166**: 11–15 (available at http://jcb.rupress.org/content/166/1/11.full).

■ First author; *see order of authors*

■ Footnotes

Most medical journals do not allow footnotes. The only exception is that some journals use footnotes to acknowledge funding or to list study group members who are not identified individually on the by-line. (However, do not assume that listing names in a footnote means that these individuals do not need to fulfil authorship criteria – *see* **by-lines**, **order of authors** and **contributorship vs. authorship** for more details on this tricky area.)

Another possible exception is if new data emerge after a paper is typeset and you want to add an update to the proofs. Rather than resetting large sections of text, or renumbering references, the journal might prefer this to appear as a footnote – although, in these days of computer typesetting, this is probably needlessly old-fashioned.

Journals of law or medical ethics, on the other hand, may positively encourage footnotes. The rule, as always, is to check a recent copy of your target journal. If footnotes are permitted, check how these should be included in a manuscript or electronic submission.

Some people use the 'Endnote' function of Word to produce reference lists, although I find dedicated bibliographic software far more efficient. If you have used either of these, check that this does not mess up an electronic submission.

■ Formatting requirements

Most journals expect submitted manuscripts to follow their sometimes exacting formatting requirements for things like references and abstract headings. While the pain of reference formatting (and reformatting) can largely be removed by using **bibliographic software**, detailed formatting does waste time if your submission is rejected and you have to reformat for another journal. A few, enlightened journals now allow authors to submit manuscripts in any reasonable format and only expect you to follow their specific instructions once your work has been accepted. Elsevier has led the charge on this, announcing 'Your Paper, Your Way' in some of its journals in 2011, although this welcome policy appears to be taking a while to reach the medical journals. You probably shouldn't try to submit your masterpiece written on parchment with purple crayon or if it is twice the journal's word limit but it is good to see that some publishers have recognised the annoyance caused to authors by reformatting and tried to reduce it.

www.elsevier.com/authors-update/story/online-submissionpeer-review/your-paper-your-way-simplifies-papers-submission

■ Freebies / 'throwaways'

Freebies (or 'throwaways') are medical newspapers or websites such as *Pulse* in the UK, and *Family Practice News* in the US. They are funded by advertising, available to large numbers of doctors and quite widely read. They often contain short, practical review or educational articles as well as news items but they virtually never carry original research and rarely accept unsolicited items. If you want to write for the freebies you should contact the editor directly with your ideas, but you should not plan to publish your research this way. However, if your findings are truly earth shattering, or you want to publicise an event or initiative, you might consider issuing a press release in the hope that it will be picked up as a news item.

■ **Funding source, role of;** *see* **sponsor, role of**

G

■ **Galley proofs**

Strictly speaking, a galley proof is the initial proof stage when text is set to the correct line width but not made up into pages. On a galley proof the text appears as a single, uninterrupted column and the figures and tables do not appear in their final positions. Electronic typesetting has made this stage almost redundant. In most cases, authors receive page proofs, which have the text laid out into the journal's usual page format with tables and figures in their correct places.

These days, the only items that sometimes appear as galley proofs are letters. This is because correspondence is usually squeezed into journals at the last minute, so the number of letters that appear in each issue will depend on how much space the articles occupy. Journal editors may therefore get authors to approve galley proofs of letters and then make up the journal pages when the rest of the issue is finalised. As letters rarely contain figures or tables, and are often short, this usually poses no problems, so you can treat them like page proofs.

For some reason, some people continue to refer to all proofs as galley proofs (or, to show how well they think they know the jargon, simply as 'galleys'). So that you do not fall into this trap (and as I'm feeling pedantic), you will find details about handling proofs under 'P' for **proofs (page proofs)**. Incidentally, as I'm being pedantic, you might like to know that the word 'galley' refers to the rectangular tray into which metal type used to be set, not an ancient ship.

■ **Gap analysis**

This technique is sometimes used by drug companies to identify publications that might support the marketing of their products. Rather than starting with a study, deciding what the findings show and publishing them, the company may identify a claim it would like to make about its product, or an audience it would like to reach with a particular message, and then go about generating publications to achieve this. In some cases this may involve designing and running new studies, which, if they answer important clinical questions, may be a good thing; but there is a risk that it can lead to dredging data in a search for evidence. However, it may result in legitimate and useful **secondary publications** (such as review articles focusing on new questions or written for different readerships). Responsible publication plans should be driven by the findings of trials designed to answer predefined and clinically relevant questions. Sometimes it is possible to pool findings or do secondary analyses in an attempt to answer other questions, but care and statistical advice are needed.

■ Ghost authors

A ghost author is somebody who qualifies for authorship but is not included in a publication's author list. The occurrence of ghosts is bad for everybody concerned. It deprives the ghost author of recognition and it misleads readers about who did the work. The most common cause of ghosts is sponsors trying to underplay their involvement in studies by limiting the number of company authors, but authors may also be omitted because of professional (academic) rivalry.

The best way to avoid ghost authors is to agree authorship criteria early in the research process. When the study is complete, the criteria should be checked to make sure that everybody who qualifies is included in preparing the publication(s).

Ghost authorship should not be confused with 'ghost writing' – a term sometimes used when a medical writer, who does not usually qualify for authorship, assists with a publication but is not acknowledged – read on for further details.

A study of ghost authorship, which looked for people who were named on a study protocol but not on the publication, found that statisticians suffered this spectral fate more often than medical writers.

Gøtzsche PC, Hróbjartsson A, Johansen HK *et al.* (2007) Ghost authorship in industry-initiated randomised trials. *PLoS Med.* **4**: e19.

■ Ghost writers

This term is sometimes applied to a professional medical writer who has not been involved with a study but who helps develop a publication – in particular, by preparing the first draft. The term is unfortunate as it implies that the writer's identity is not revealed. However, getting help from a professional writer is no more shameful than getting advice from a professional statistician and the involvement of a writer should not be confused with questions about competing interests or of sponsors trying to exert undue influence over publications. It is therefore important that the writer and their source of funding should be identified (usually in the **acknowledgements** section) which effectively exorcises the paper.

The question of whether a writer qualifies as an author is a matter for judgement. Unless a writer has contributed to the interpretation of the data and is prepared to take public responsibility for the research (not just responsibility for how the publication was prepared) they will not meet the **International Committee of Medical Journal Editors' (ICMJE)** authorship criteria and therefore, in most journals, they should not appear on the **by-line**. However, a few journals (e.g. *Neurology*) argue that the preparation of a draft is, in itself, an act of interpretation, and prefer the writer to be listed as an author, or at least as a contributor (*see* **acknowledgements**).

How much data interpretation the writer does will depend on how the paper is developed. Both **Good Publication Practice (GPP)** for company-sponsored publications and the **European Medical Writers Assocation (EMWA)** guidelines recommend that a draft should not be prepared until an **outline** has been agreed with the named authors. If a detailed outline and **key messages** are established from discussions with the named authors, the writer may have only a limited role in deciding how data are presented or interpreted. However, if a writer takes a more active role, for example by searching and synthesising the literature for a review article or for the introduction or discussion sections of a primary paper, the writer's contribution may merit authorship.

The EMWA guidelines for medical writers and GPP contain practical recommendations for the appropriate use of medical writers in developing publications.

Jacobs A and Wager E (2005) European Medical Writers Association (EMWA) guidelines on the role of medical writers in developing medical publications. *Curr Med Res Opin.* **21**: 317–21. www.emwa.org/documents/about_us/EMWAguidelines.pdf

Battisti W, Wager E, Baltzer L *et al.* (2015) Good Publication Practice for communicating company-sponsored medical research: GPP3. *Ann Intern Med.* **163**: doi:10.7326/M15-0288.

See also Chapter 4 'Working with a medical writer' (pp. 19–21).

■ Gift authorship; *see guest authors*

■ Gold Open Access

Gold is used to denote journals that make articles freely available to readers on their own website and also allow their wide reuse, usually via a **Creative Commons licence**. This means that authors (and others) can post copies on their personal website. (Other colours of Open Access are green and diamond.)

■ Good Publication Practice (GPP, GPP2 and GPP3)

This is a set of guidelines that aim to encourage the responsible reporting of company-sponsored research. Although the GPP guidelines refer to both the **International Committee of Medical Journal Editors' (ICMJE)** guidelines and the **CONSORT** statement, they go beyond both of these, in particular by including detailed recommendations about the role of professional medical writers and relations between doctors and drug company sponsors – something about which most other guidelines are silent.

The original GPP guidelines arose from a meeting in 1999 between journal editors, academic investigators and drug company personnel. One area of particular concern for both the editors and the academics was **publication bias**, i.e. the tendency for favourable findings to be published more than negative ones. GPP therefore called on companies to endeavour to publish the results of all clinical trials of marketed products. GPP also provided guidance on ways to avoid covert **redundant publication**, such as clear study identification. The first version of GPP was published in 2003.

GPP was endorsed by several drug companies, supported by a number of communication agencies, and included in the 'Instructions to contributors' of *The BMJ* and **BioMed Central** journals.

The original GPP guidelines were revised after extensive consultation coordinated by the **International Society for Medical Publication Professionals (ISMPP)**, resulting in the publication of GPP2 in late 2009 and GPP3 in 2015. Newer versions include guidance on publication planning and 10 principles of good practice that should apply to all publications, not just those describing commercially sponsored research (*see* Appendix 4). As I have been involved from the beginning, and in case you are interested in the evolution of the guidelines, I'm indulging my pride by listing all three versions. I'm horribly biased, but I reckon they are essential reading for anybody involved with publications that report company-sponsored research.

Wager E, Field EA and Grossman L (2003) Good Publication Practice for pharmaceutical companies. *Curr Med Res Opin.* **19**: 149–54.

Graf C, Battisti WP, Bridges D *et al.* (2009) Good Publication Practice for communicating company sponsored medical research: GPP2. *BMJ.* **339**: b4330.

Battisti WP, Wager E, Baltzer L *et al.* (2015) Good Publication Practice for communicating company-sponsored medical research: GPP3. *Ann Intern Med.* **163**: doi:10.7326/M15-0288.

If you want to know more about how GPP developed, you can read my blog post about it.

Liz Wager (August 2015): GPP3 – thoughts on becoming a guideline grandmother. http://blogs.bmj.com/bmj/2015/08/26/liz-wager-gpp3-thoughts-on-becoming-a-guideline-grandmother/

■ Graphs

See also **figures**. If you use graphs a lot, and enjoy fiddling about with this sort of thing, it may be worth investing in specialist software to produce them for your publication. However, although such packages are versatile and powerful, they take a while to learn and it is easy to forget what all the features do unless you use them frequently. I therefore find it easier, quicker (and, if you are counting your time, cheaper) to get graphs prepared by a professional illustrator or designer. Such people can produce high quality figures in formats acceptable to journals.

Green Open Access

Green Open Access might be regarded, by some, as not really proper Open Access. It denotes journals that allow authors to self-archive their work (i.e. to post it on an institutional or personal website), but that don't give immediate free access to readers via the journal (or publisher's) website. Articles published in this type of journal are therefore slightly less easy for readers to access than those appearing in Gold Open Access journals. However, search engines such as Google Scholar do make it possible to find alternative versions of articles, so this may enable readers to find the full text. If you want to post your article on your own (or an institutional) website, do check the small print of the licensing agreement, as some publishers do not allow authors to post the published PDFs but only the final manuscript.

Group authorship

Authorship by a group (rather than a list of individuals) is sometimes suggested, perhaps in the hope of avoiding difficult decisions about author order and number. Although this may seem like a neat solution, it has some drawbacks. For a start, some journals won't allow it, so check your target journal. Secondly, databases such as Medline often don't handle group names very cleverly, so they may be mis-cited. There is even evidence that studies with only group authors are cited less often than those with real people on the by-line.[1]

Acknowledging a group in addition to individuals is generally a better idea, but you still need to check your target journal. Some journals will allow Author N, Writer A on behalf of the CHUMMY Study Group and will print a list of members of the study group. Others insist that all listed group members meet authorship criteria – which rather defeats the object.

You can see the effects of different journal policies in the versions of the **Good Publication Practice (GPP)** guidelines. GPP2 was published in *The BMJ*, which allowed the inclusion of the words 'for the International Society for Medical Publication Professionals' to be included after the list of individual authors. GPP3 was published in the *Annals of Internal Medicine* which only allowed ISMPP to be mentioned in the acknowledgements but not in the by-line.

Since 2008, Medline has allowed collaborators to be listed in the database and recognises that these are different from authors. It notes that 'When a group name is included as an author, the respective group member names appearing in the article will be acknowledged as collaborators but not associated with authorship'.

ICMJE notes 'When submitting a manuscript authored by a group, the corresponding author should specify the group name if one exists, and clearly identify the group members who can take credit and responsibility for the work as authors. The byline of the article identifies who is directly responsible for the manuscript, and MEDLINE lists as authors whichever names appear on the byline. If the byline includes a group name, MEDLINE will list the names of individual group members who are authors or who are collaborators, sometimes called non-author contributors, if there is a note associated with the byline clearly stating that the individual names are elsewhere in the paper and whether those names are authors or collaborators'.

www.nlm.nih.gov/pubs/techbull/ma08/ma08_collaborators.html

www.icmje.org/recommendations

1 Dickersin K, Scherer R, Suci ES *et al.* (2002) Problems with indexing and citation of articles with group authorship. *JAMA.* **287**: 2772–4.

■ Guarantor

Journals that have adopted the **contributorship** system (i.e. those that list individuals' contributions to a piece of work) may ask that one contributor guarantees the project's integrity. The idea behind this is that individuals may have specialist roles within complex studies. It is therefore unreasonable to expect the statistician to justify the choice of dose, or for a clinician to explain why a certain statistical test was used. However, if each person takes responsibility for only part of the study somebody needs to guarantee the integrity of the overall project. Check your target journal's instructions (or a recent issue) to see if you need to nominate a guarantor. Conventionally, this person will often be the first or **last author**, but there are no rules about this. The 2013 revision of the ICMJE guidelines rather mysteriously dropped any mention of guarantors but emphasises the **accountability** of all authors.

■ Guest authors / gift authorship

Guests are people who are invited to be listed as authors although they do not meet authorship criteria (or fulfil the criteria less well than others who are not included). Guests are usually included for their prestige, in the hope that adding their name will increase a publication's chance of acceptance or its impact on readers. They may also be included to curry favour or for mutual CV enlargement. The latter occurs in competitive academic fields, or those in which promotion or tenure depends on the length (rather than the quality) of a person's publication list, when researchers add colleagues' names to papers on the understanding that the colleagues will do the same for them. Drug companies may be tempted to offer guest authorship to eminent opinion leaders in the hope that this will endear them to the company and add credibility to the research, although, if the practice is disclosed, it could have the opposite effect.

Whatever the motive, guest authorship should be discouraged, since it presents a dishonest picture of how a study was performed, is likely to irritate the 'real' authors, and may increase the likelihood of deserving authors being omitted.

However, the habit may be hard to break if there is a strong tradition of the professor being included in every publication from his or her department. It is a brave junior researcher who is prepared to question this practice even when armed with clear guidance from the target journal and the **International Committee of Medical Journal Editors' (ICMJE)** criteria, which state that obtaining funding or general supervision of a research group, by themselves, are not automatic qualifications for authorship. The trend for journals to list individuals' contributions rather than just their names (i.e. **contributorship**) may help discourage guest authorship, since it may help readers and editors to identify guests. However, with the traditional author **by-line** it is usually impossible for anybody outside the research team to distinguish deserving authors from guests. Some journals require authors to sign a statement that they meet the ICMJE criteria; however, people prepared to accept gift authorship are often quite happy to make a dishonest declaration so this probably has little effect.

Institutional authorship policies, in particular outlawing the practice of always including the head of department, are likely to be more effective. But, sadly, few academic institutions have such policies in place. Junior researchers seeking ammunition may find the COPE guidelines on authorship (available at www. publicationethics.org.uk) helpful – but I am probably biased, as I am one of the authors (and not a guest).

H

◼ Hanging Committee

This is the name of a *BMJ* committee that used to be the final judge of whether submissions were accepted. It got its name from the committee at London's Royal Academy that selects pictures to hang on the walls at its summer exhibition (although to rejected authors its actions may have resembled capital punishment).

In other journals the **editorial board** may serve a similar function. At *The Lancet*, papers are discussed by all editors at a weekly meeting (but it doesn't have a funny name).

◼ Hijacked journals; *see* cloned journals

■ Hot topics

Journal acceptance rates are, by definition, averages. One way of increasing your chance of acceptance is by researching your **target journal** well. This means not only knowing the types of articles it publishes, but reading the most recent issues to see if any themes or 'hot topics' emerge. Unfortunately, you can't usually plan your research to coincide with a journal editor's latest interest; however, given a choice of two rather similar journals, only one of which has published papers on a similar theme to yours, it is a good idea to select that journal.

However, you should not confuse hot topics with similar studies. Companies usually have to perform two or three large (so-called Phase III) studies in order to license a new drug. Very often these pivotal studies have virtually identical designs. If a journal has already published the results of one pivotal trial, it is unlikely to accept another. Since such trials often take place in different locations, a better strategy is to consider the journal's geographic reach and readership, for example submitting a North American study to a US journal, and a European one to a European journal.

■ House style

Virtually all journals (except a few electronic ones that do not invest in any copy editing) will impose their own (so-called 'house') style on your article before publication. House style includes spelling options (e.g. US versus UK, -ise versus -ize), conventions on abbreviations (e.g. how e.g. is punctuated) and typographic style for headings. There is no point in resisting this or trying to revert to your original version on the proofs. However, there is also no need to try to make your submission conform exactly to your target journal's style by using the same format for headings, etc. Although this might make you look keen and show that you have researched the journal thoroughly, most publishers actually prefer to receive simple text without fancy styles, as word processing codes usually have to be replaced with typesetting commands, so heavily formatted text may actually slow the process down. That is not to say that you should not follow the 'Instructions to authors', especially the preferred reference style (which will be simple if you have invested in **bibliographic software**), but, having done this, you need not try to make your typescript look exactly like a published paper.

House wine and house dressing are outside the scope of this book but may, if used judiciously, ease the publication process especially if they ensure that authors have time to get to know one another and discuss their publications in congenial surroundings. Many publication problems arise through lack of communication, so the more everybody can talk and get to know other team members, the smoother the process is likely to be.

■ Hybrid journals

These are journals that allow authors to make individual articles free to readers, if they pay an **article processing charge**, but which charge readers a subscription to read articles by authors who have not paid for the **Open Access** option. Most big publishers do this; see, for example:

- Oxford Open (www.oxfordjournals.org/en/oxford-open/index.html)
- Springer Open Choice (www.springer.com/gp/open-access/springer-open-choice)
- Wiley OnlineOpen (http://olabout.wiley.com/WileyCDA/Section/id-406241.html).

This practice has been condemned by some universities as 'double dipping' since these institutions end up paying both the journal subscriptions for their libraries and the article processing charges for their researchers. See, for example, www.rluk.ac.uk/about-us/blog/the-costs-of-double-dipping/.

I

■ ICMJE; *see* International Committee of Medical Journal Editors

■ Image manipulation; *see* figures

■ Impact factors

Impact factors (IFs) are a measure of how often a journal's papers get cited. This is not a bad idea in itself, but, unfortunately, many academic institutions attach undue importance to IFs and use them to assess the importance of individual publications or researchers, which they were never designed to do. Some journal editors also get a bit over-excited about their IF. So, although it is tempting to say you should ignore them, you need to understand their misuse.

Official journal IFs are published each year by Thomson Reuters, a commercial company which selects the journals on which it bestows this honour and charges publishers large amounts for each year's Journal Citation Reports. For details see http://wokinfo.com/products_tools/analytical/jcr/.

In response to the rise of **predatory journals** other companies have sprung up offering alternative (or bogus) IFs, so do check the exact name and don't assume that all IFs (or similar sounding things) are equal.

IFs are calculated by dividing the number of times a journal is cited in a given year by the number of full papers it has published in the previous 2 years. Letters and abstracts are not included in the denominator, although, of course, they may be cited – so journals that publish a lot of these may have inflated IFs. Journals are grouped into subjects (e.g. dermatology, general medicine) and ranked by IF. The prestigious general journals (e.g. *NEJM*, *The Lancet*) have much higher IFs than specialist journals.

While it is quite interesting to see how journals rank, there is probably only a very rough correlation between the whole journal's IF and the impact of a single publication. Some papers in the highest IF journals are never cited at all, while others become classics, so the average is a pretty crude statistic. Nevertheless, some universities rate the output of a department or researcher by multiplying the number of their publications by the IF of the journal in which they appeared. In some countries an individual needs a certain number of such publication 'points' before s/he can be appointed to the next grade (e.g. a professorship). This has the unfortunate effect of increasing the attractions of **guest authorship** (i.e. including colleagues' names on papers although they have contributed little or nothing to the research) and of making the IF the most important criterion for academics when selecting a journal. This abuse of the IF has been roundly criticised by the *San Francisco Declaration on Research Assessment* (or DORA) which has been endorsed by some, more enlightened, universities and funders.

Although the IF is one factor to bear in mind, it is a mistake to forget about the journal's readership, acceptance rate, time to publication, etc. when selecting a **target journal**. Great emphasis on IF can lead to academics insisting on submitting papers to journals that are unlikely to accept them, which often wastes time. It may also cause disagreements among authors if some want to hold out for the highest IF while others (or the study's sponsors) are more interested in a rapid publication or some other criterion. Remember that journals can't have an IF until they have been published for at least 3 years so new journals, even from reputable publishers, don't have them (e.g. at the time of writing the third edition, *Lancet Psychiatry*, launched in 2014, didn't have one).

The current IF listings are only available at a high price from Web of Knowledge, which guards its copyright fiercely. However, you can often discover an individual journal's IF from its website or by making an enquiry to its editorial office.

Journal IFs vary between specialties, so if you are considering more than one target audience it is unwise to try to compare journals from different areas. (For example, if you wanted to publish a study on childhood asthma, you should consider the IFs of paediatrics journals separately from those for respiratory medicine – the rank order is a more reliable guide to a journal's influence than the numerical value of its IF – although, of course, if your sole aim is to choose the journal with the highest IF then there's no harm shopping around.)

Sadly, there is a correlation between IF and rejection rate – hence picking the journal with the highest IF will often increase your chance of rejection.

If co-authors cannot agree on a target journal, they might agree to the following compromise. The first choice journal will be one with a high IF (thus probably also a high rejection rate) but also a relatively rapid time to reject (e.g. one that rejects a large proportion of submissions after **in-house review**). If you get rejected, honour will have been satisfied, but you won't have wasted too much time. Everyone must agree (before submission to the first journal) that, if the paper is rejected by the first journal, it will be submitted (straightaway, and without further prolonged discussion) to a second journal with a greater chance of acceptance.

If all authors are determined to get the most IF points from a paper, you can work your way down the ranking until your paper is accepted. But, even the most assessment-conscious academic usually gets disheartened after a couple of rejections, and it gets harder to revise a paper the further you are from doing the research, so this strategy could, paradoxically, result in everybody getting fed up and the paper never being published (so no IF points for anybody). It is far better to agree your target audience, research your target carefully, be realistic about your chances of acceptance and regard the journal's IF as a side issue.

If you already know the IFs of all the journals in your specialty or can quote any IF to two decimal places, this is a strong indication that you are seriously over-stressed in your struggle for promotion or your department's research assessment exercise and need to take a holiday.

Getting clever with IFs

Some editors get very competitive about their journal's IF and have even been known to try to inflate their figures by devious means. For example, a few editors have been caught demanding that authors include a certain number of citations to their own journal. While this is not considered good form among journal editors, authors should take note. Since journal editors like citations to their own journal, you might curry favour by including as many as possible. Don't overdo this, or include irrelevant references just because they come from the target journal, but it probably won't do any harm if you slip in a couple of citations of review articles or previous studies from the journal in your introduction. Apart from raising the journal's IF, including citations from previous publications is also a sign that you have selected your target journal with care, and may provide some reasons why the editor should publish your work, especially if it complements something the journal has already published.

Smith R (1997) Journal accused of manipulating impact factor. *BMJ*. **314**: 463.

The Thomson Reuters impact factor (1994). http://wokinfo.com/essays/impact-factor/

EASE statement on inappropriate use of impact factors (2007). www.ease.org.uk/publications/impact-factor-statement

San Francisco Declaration on Research Assessment (2012). http://am.ascb.org/dora/

Beall J (2013) Look out for bogus impact factor companies. Scholarly Open Access blog. http://scholarlyoa.com/2013/08/06/bogus-impact-factor-companies/

■ IMRAD structure

Acronym for Introduction, Methods, Results and Discussion, used to describe the conventional structure of a scientific paper.

■ Indexing

Publishing in a journal that is indexed in the major databases will increase the chances of your paper being identified in literature searches. The most widely used database is **Medline**, produced by the US National Library of Medicine and available (free of charge) at www.ncbi.nlm.nih.gov/PubMed.

However, by no means all medical journals are included on Medline, and non-English language publications are particularly poorly represented. Other databases such as Embase (www.elsevier.com/solutions/embase) and Scopus (www.elsevier.com/solutions/scopus) include more titles, but charge a search fee so they tend to be available only at libraries and academic institutions, thus limiting access to well-funded researchers. Choosing a journal that is included in Medline or is on **PubMed Central** may therefore increase the accessibility of your publication.

Journals often ask for key words to help the indexing services classify articles correctly; it is therefore worth spending a few moments to select the best ones – *see* **key words** for more details.

While Medline is the primary global medical database, others may also be relevant for your research, such as LILACS for journals from Latin America and the Caribbean (http://lilacs.bvsalud.org/en/) and CINAHL for the nursing and allied health literature (https://health.ebsco.com/products/cinahl-plus-with-full-text).

■ Informal review

In your efforts to involve all the right **(key) people** and to jump through the hoops created by peer review it is easy to overlook informal review. Much of this book is about making sure a publication is reviewed by the right people at the right time, but you should also consider adding some extra, informal review steps. If parts of the submission are written by non-native English speakers, or even if they are written by several native speakers with different styles, it may be helpful to get a review from a native-speaking writer or editor. If you have access to information specialists or librarians they may be prepared to check your references. People outside your subject area such as husbands, wives or even cooperative children can sometimes spot flaws in the logic or ways in which a paper could be made more accessible to a wider audience. Lay people are good at asking probing questions such as 'Why does this matter?' or 'Why did you do this?' which can help structure the introduction or discussion. *See also* Table 1.1, p. 4.

The secret of using informal review is to give very clear instructions. Explain to the potential reviewer exactly why you are asking them to read the paper and what you would like them to do, and give them a deadline. The timing of informal review is also important. There is no point doing a final check for grammar and spelling on sections that are likely to be rewritten. If you approach colleagues or investigators outside the writing group for their input you must also be clear about what rewards they can (and should not) expect – in particular, make it clear that their contribution will not lead to authorship if that is the case. If informal reviewers have been particularly helpful you should consider mentioning them in the **acknowledgements**.

For more information see the chapter on informal review in:

Wager E, Godlee F and Jefferson T (2002) *How to Survive Peer Review*. BMJ Books, London.

■ Ingelfinger rule

The principle that journals will not consider work that has been published elsewhere is sometimes termed the Ingelfinger rule after Franz J Ingelfinger, the Editor of the *New England Journal of Medicine*, who promoted this in 1969.

Angell M and Kassirer JP (1991) The Ingelfinger Rule revisited. *N Engl J Med.* **325**: 1371–3.

See also **prior publication**.

■ In-house review

Journals that employ several editors and receive many submissions often reject a considerable proportion of manuscripts after in-house review. This means that average times to rejection are shorter than those for acceptance. *See* **review process** and Chapter 3 'How long will it take?' (pp. 13–17) for more details.

The purpose of in-house review is to reduce the burden on external reviewers by sifting out submissions that are unsuitable for a particular journal. Editors rejecting papers during in-house review are most concerned about whether the findings are likely to interest their readers and whether the article fits the journal's scope rather than whether it follows reporting guidelines or the study was well executed. Editors (especially full-time ones) are generally not experts on your particular topic but do know what sort of articles they like to publish. If you are rejected after in-house review you therefore do not receive detailed criticism of your research or suggestions on how to improve your paper, but usually just a note saying 'sorry, it's not for us'. If you have failed to excite the editor sufficiently to warrant external review it probably means you have selected the wrong journal, so there is little point in appealing, and it is usually better to follow your **back-up plan** and submit to another journal. As *The BMJ* notes, 'If the editors … have decided that your paper is not sufficiently interesting or important for *BMJ* readers, there may be no point in trying to appeal'. However, you might consider revising your paper and your **cover letter** to make sure you have explained why your research was interesting and important in the hope that you can convince another editor of its merits.

■ Initials; *see names*

■ In press; *see unpublished data*

■ Institutional repositories

Many universities have created online repositories for work published by their staff and students. These may be useful to provide access to the full text for readers if the work is published in a **Green** (rather than **Gold**) **Open Access** journal – *see* these entries for more details. Authors should check their institution's policies as well as the journal's policy to understand what should and shouldn't be posted.

One problem with institutional repositories and **personal websites** is that they usually contain the first published version (or sometimes the accepted version before copy editing), and may not indicate if an article is subsequently corrected or retracted. The **CrossMark** system has been developed to reduce this problem and identify the updated version maintained by the publisher. If repositories include PDFs with the CrossMark logo, readers can click on the logo to check for updates.

Institutional repositories may also contain dissertations and theses which sometimes cause problems when journals screen submissions using text-matching software because they may appear as redundant publications. However, most editors would regard such a match as a false positive, as inclusion of material in a thesis does not usually prevent publication in a journal. (But, of course, if somebody has copied material from another person's unpublished thesis, the software helpfully highlights such **plagiarism**.)

A handy tool to identify institutional repositories is the OpenDOAR directory (www.opendoar.org/).

■ Instructions to authors (contributors)

However helpful this book might be, there is no substitute for reading your target journal's instructions. These are available on journal or publisher websites, so you do not even need to leave the comfort of your office or lab. Read the instructions as soon as you select your target journal, then again before you prepare the submission package.

It is easy to get irritated by journal **formatting requirements**, especially if you are already in a bad mood because your paper has been rejected by your first choice journal. If necessary, go and have a cup of coffee (or something stronger), or wait until you are feeling calmer, then tackle them like you would an exam question, making sure you have answered every point. If possible, get into a frame of mind that allows you to take pedantic pride in getting every little detail right. This will not guarantee acceptance but it should make a good impression on the editor and reviewers and certainly will not damage your chances.

If you really can't be bothered to format (or reformat) your article right now you could select a journal that doesn't require formatting until after acceptance – a policy introduced recently by some Elsevier journals and *PeerJ*, which I predict will be popular with many authors.

Fennell C and Barrie R (2014) Your Paper, Your Way and the reviewing process. Elsevier blog. www.elsevier.com/reviewers-update/story/innovation-in-publishing/your-paper,-your-way-and-the-reviewing-process

■ Internal review

Virtually everybody has a boss or employer who will need to see papers or abstracts before submission so, unless all the authors are self-employed and self-funded, internal review is inevitable. In the case of big drug companies, this internal review may be complex and time-consuming. When you are planning a publication, try to find out what review steps will be needed and roughly how long they will take. Large companies usually have standard times (or targets) for review. It is also important to establish at what stage the various reviews should take place, and which can take place in parallel (to save time) rather than sequentially.

If you are collating comments you will also need to understand which changes take precedence. Some companies have a formal hierarchy for this, which, although it looks bureaucratic, is actually very helpful for an external writer or editor who then knows that, for example, changes suggested by the global legal department are sacrosanct, while comments from the Ruritanian medical department can be ignored if they clash with others. **GPP3** recommends that companies' commercial functions (i.e. sales and marketing departments) should not be involved in publication review or **approval**.

If you are designing a review process, it is best to aim for a pyramid structure, which involves lots of people at the early (e.g. outline) stages, and gradually fewer and fewer people (apart, of course, from the authors) at the later stages.

If you are writing up sponsored research, check your **contract** or investigators' agreement to see whether the sponsor needs to review any planned submissions (they usually do), and, if so, how much time they need for this (60 days is not uncommon). Even if this is not stated in your contract, it is courteous to inform the sponsor about any planned publications.

■ International Clinical Trials Registry Platform (ICTRP)

This is a portal, maintained by the World Health Organization (WHO), that allows searches across several trial registers. It does not constitute a trial register itself but gathers information from a number of national and other registers. The WHO established quality criteria for registers to be included and such registers are referred to as primary registers. The list of primary registers is relevant to publication planners because the **ICMJE** specifies these registers in its requirement for trial registration.

www.who.int/ictrp/en/

■ International Committee of Medical Journal Editors (ICMJE)

This is an influential group of medical journal editors who periodically issue guidance and pronouncements that have been endorsed by a much wider group of journals. The best known of these guidelines was, until 2013, called the 'Uniform requirements for manuscripts submitted to biomedical journals' and you will still see this name (or URM) in outdated references. It now goes under the rather unwieldy title of 'Recommendations for the conduct, reporting, editing, and publication of scholarly work in medical journals' (it is available at www.icmje.org).

The ICMJE's Recommendations and other statements provide much useful information about topics such as authorship and overlapping publications that are often not covered in individual journal instructions, so they are worth reading even if you plan to publish in a journal that has not formally endorsed them. The location of the group's first meeting (in 1978) gave its name to the Vancouver style of references in which citations are numbered in the text and listed by their order of appearance in the reference list. However, 'Vancouver style' is a generic term and there are endless subtle variations on this theme such as how many authors are listed before you use *et al.*, the punctuation of authors' names and whether journal names are abbreviated.

Considering how easy it is to format references using **bibliographic software** there is really no excuse for not following the exact style of your target journal.

Similarly, the ICMJE Recommendations do not tell you exactly how to structure an **abstract**, whether **key words** are used, etc. Although it should not matter, it does not do any harm to show that you have researched your target journal (and are not on the rebound from another) by formatting your submission precisely to the individual journal's style.

As noted on its own website, the ICMJE is 'not an open membership organization' and its exclusive nature has sometimes been criticised (especially by journal editors who haven't been invited). The current (August 2015) members of the ICMJE are the editors of:

- *Annals of Internal Medicine*
- *The BMJ (British Medical Journal)*
- *Canadian Medical Association Journal*
- *Chinese Medical Journal*
- *Ethiopian Journal of Health Sciences*
- *JAMA (The Journal of the American Medical Association)*
- *Nederlands Tijdschrift voor Geneeskunde (Dutch Journal of Medicine)*
- *The New England Journal of Medicine*
- *New Zealand Journal of Medicine*
- *Revista Médica de Chile*
- *The Lancet.*

■ International Society for Medical Publication Professionals (ISMPP)

While medical writers organisations (such as **AMWA**) date back to the 1940s, publication planners didn't have their own society until 2005, when ISMPP (pronounced 'iz-map') was founded. Since then it has grown to include over 1400 members and has well-attended annual meetings in the USA and Europe. If you have a publications role in a drug or medical device company, or a specialist agency, you should consider joining so you can meet other people working in the area and keep abreast of new developments. ISMPP has also developed a credentialing system, to recognise **Certified Medical Publication Professionals (CMPP)** so you can even get letters after your name if you pass their exam. If you are reading this book in preparation for the CMPP exam – good luck, and I hope it is helpful! For more information see www.ismpp.org.

■ Investigators' agreements

This is an ideal place to set out the publication policy, including data ownership and authorship criteria. Starting to discuss the publication strategy in the early stages of the research process is helpful, even if many details cannot be finalised until the data have been analysed. Thinking about the publication(s) before you start a study may also help to plan your research and ensure that you generate publishable results. Although the small print and legal language may be daunting, you should read agreements carefully before you sign them to make sure you are comfortable with proposals for data access and how publications will be developed. Check for any restrictions on publication. Sponsors should not be allowed to veto publications but it is reasonable for them to require review of manuscripts before submission, for example to make sure there are no intellectual property issues (such as disclosures that might affect a patent filing). *See* **contracts** and **publication agreements** for more details.

■ ISRCTN (International Standard Randomised Controlled Trial Number)

This trial register was originally set up by a commercial publisher but was later transferred to a not-for-profit foundation. Although it meets the International Committee of Medical Journal Editors' requirements for an acceptable place to register clinical trials it does not include a results database and does not meet the requirements of **FDAAA** (the US law passed in 2007 which, effectively, required most trials to be registered on the US website **ClinicalTrials.gov**). Lacking government money (unlike ClinicalTrials.gov), ISRCTN has to charge a small administrative fee to registrants (although it is free to search), which is another reason why it may be doomed to obscurity. Which is a shame, because although ClinicalTrials.gov currently does an excellent job, the effective monopoly of a single register funded by one government (in this case the US) is a bit scary and some people would prefer trial registration to be controlled by a more neutral, international organisation.

J

■ Journal cascades and consortia

Publishers whose journals include both highly selective and less selective titles realise that it benefits both them and the authors if submissions rejected by one journal can be passed, along with the reviewer comments, to other journals in the group. Several publishers have even established journals obviously aimed at benefiting from the trickle down from their big-name (and high-rejection-rate) journals (e.g. *The Lancet* specialist journals and *BMJ Open*).

When choosing an ambitious target journal (i.e. one with a high rejection rate) it is always a good idea to plan a second target, and if you pick two within a cascade you may not have to wait for the second journal to review your article, especially if the peer reviewers for the original journal weren't too negative. However, you do not have to accept the publisher's suggestion to cascade your article. The cascade offered by the publisher might be a bad strategy if the second journal in the group is much less suitable for your work (or less prestigious) than another journal from a different publisher. For example, the gap in impact factors between selective and less selective journals in a group may be considerable (e.g. impact factors were 17.4 for *The BMJ* but only 2.3 for *BMJ Open* in 2015, while *SpringerPlus*, which is offered as a cascade to many Springer journals, did not have an impact factor), so authors might want to try some mid-ranking journals first, rather than those suggested by the publisher.

If possible, check the options for cascading before you submit, and discuss this with your co-authors so that everybody agrees the strategy for the second target (as you often have to indicate whether you wish to be included in a cascade when you submit to your first target journal).

Cascades generally refer to groups of journals produced by a single publisher such as Elsevier's Article Transfer Service (www.elsevier.com/authors/journal-authors/submit-your-paper). However, a similar system also works in a few disciplines in the form of journal consortia. These are informal groupings (without financial ties) that agree to share reviewer comments. One of the longest established is the Neuroscience Peer Review Consortium (http://nprc.incf.org/) established in 2008, which now includes almost 50 journals.

See also **reviewers' comments**.

■ Journal choice

This is the single most important decision within your publication strategy. Choice of journal will affect:

- what formats are available
- your chance of acceptance
- how long you have to wait for a decision
- the length of time from acceptance to publication
- who will read your work (at least initially)
- who will have access to your work via the web
- how your work is published (i.e. electronically, in print, or both)
- how your work is presented (e.g. how much copy editing is done at the journal)
- the visual appearance of your work (e.g. page layout, journal house style)
- how your research is perceived.

In a truly rational and scientific world, authors would sit down with a list of all available journals and information about all these variables and calculate the correct answer (and I would probably be out of a job because nobody would need my advice or want to read this book). However (and luckily for me), real life is messy, it is often hard to get all the information you need and, even faced with good evidence, humans may make subjective decisions. If you, your co-authors and other key players can agree on the choice of target journal (and, very importantly, also on the second choice) amicably over a few beers or a coffee, that is fine. But for a more logical (and beverage-free) approach follow these steps.

1. Agree the **target audience** for your publication – aim to identify their discipline, degree of specialisation and location, e.g. European family doctors with an interest in research, North American cardiologists or Japanese medical students.
2. Scan the library, the internet and reference sections of related papers to develop a 'long-list' of possible journals likely to be read by your target audience.
3. Read the journals' 'Instructions to authors' to check whether these journals meet your needs in terms of the **article formats** and any other restrictions such as article length. Eliminate any that do not.
4. Scan recent issues of possible journals to get an idea of the scope, coverage and **hot topics**. Do not rely on the journal **title** to determine this.
5. Decide how important the following factors are to you and the other **key players**, not forgetting the research sponsor:
    *   speed of publication
    *   journal reputation (e.g. **impact factor**)
    *   publication medium (print or electronic)
    *   accessibility (e.g. **indexing, Open Access journals**).

Ideally, you should be able to agree on a ranking for all four factors; however, if different parties have different **expectations** (e.g. the sponsor wants to publish as quickly as possible but the first author wants to aim for the journal with the highest impact factor), you should try to agree on the top two and seek a strategy that can satisfy both.

6. Gather as much information as you can on these criteria (or, at least on your top two). You will probably already know how the journal is published (print, web, etc.) and it is relatively easy to discover how accessible it is (e.g. whether it is **Open Access**, or is included in **Medline** or **PubMed Central**). It can be more difficult to discover how long journals take to reach decisions and to publish – *see* **decision times** and **lead time** for more details. Check recent issues in case the journal publishes submission and acceptance dates for articles – these are probably more reliable than targets mentioned in general information.

    Remember that the actual time to publication will depend not only on the speed of processing at your first target journal, but also on whether it accepts your paper. You therefore need to consider your chance of acceptance. *See* **acceptance rates** for more details.

    Reputation or prestige is, by definition, a subjective judgement, of which the **impact factor** is an imperfect measure. Asking colleagues or people who work in your field what they think of different journals is probably more useful. You should also gather incidental information that might affect your decision, such as having good contacts with the editor or members of the **editorial board**, knowing that the journal plans a theme issue that coincides with your interests, or seeing that the journal has recently published a related study.

7. At last, you will be in a position to draw up your short-list. You should have identified some journals that are likely to reach your target audience, accept the type of publication you have in mind and meet your other criteria to various extents. You should tabulate this information and share it with your co-authors and any other **key players** who will have to make the decision. If you have succeeded in getting agreement on your priorities (step 5) it should be a relatively simple task to select the journal that best meets everybody's needs, with a runner-up as second choice. Lastly, if you are selecting journals for several projects (e.g. to create a product publication strategy), try to spread your choices over several journals and avoid submitting two similar studies (e.g. a North American and a European pivotal Phase III trial) to the same journal. If you have money but lack the time or inclination to research target journals yourself you can purchase information from communication agencies or specialist companies offering publication planning tools such as **DataVision** and **PubStrat**. However, while these services are often comprehensive, including lots of titles, they can only ever provide a list of journal 'vital statistics' which can't fully substitute for actually looking at recent issues and seeing what kind of articles a journal publishes.

■ Journalists; *see media relations*

■ JULIET; *see SHERPA/JULIET*

K

■ Key message(s)

Every publication should have a message, or perhaps two. This message (or messages) should be discussed and agreed among the authors. If an external writer is brought in to help develop a publication, the key message is one of the most important parts of the **brief**, and something to be discussed before writing begins.

Defining your key message before you start to write will help to focus your writing and, in particular, know which details should be stressed, and which can be omitted. In this respect publications are different from the reports written for regulatory agencies, which must contain every detail of the research. Authors and writers need to exercise scientific and moral judgement in choosing what data to include in a publication. The distinction between a persuasive and focused paper and a biased or unrepresentative one is a fine one, and you should not let enthusiasm for your message slip over into 'spin'. However, it is a mistake to imagine that the perfect scientific paper is one without a message since such papers are likely to confuse and bore readers.

As a scientist or clinician you are entitled to hold opinions about what your findings mean, and you are expected to express them, especially in the discussion section. If you are preparing a publication jointly, or several authors are preparing different publications, it is very important that all contributors agree on the key messages so that their writing has some chance of hanging together to form a consistent whole, and so that different papers from the same project do not overlap too much.

Do not make the mistake of confusing the topic (or title) with the key message. For example, the topic of a study might be the safety of Wunderdrug in patients with diabetes. This tells you about the study but does not provide sufficient focus for writing it up. A message, like a sentence, needs a verb (i.e. a word indicating action). Thus, the message might be 'Patients taking Wunderdrug have fewer hypoglycaemic episodes than patients taking Glucoglop'. Similarly, for an article about the pharmacodynamics of two treatments, the message might be 'Speedotab has a faster onset of action than Whizzopill'.

Further judgement is needed in deciding how many publications should be derived from a single piece of research. For clear communication, and to keep within journal stipulations on length, each paper should have no more than two messages. If you and your co-authors believe there are three or more messages, you should consider splitting the publication, but be careful to avoid **redundant publication** and **salami science**. Some studies divide quite naturally into sections such as efficacy and **economic (health outcomes) evaluations**. Similarly, secondary (post hoc) analyses may be best presented as separate, secondary papers – but, in this case, make sure the main paper is referenced and be transparent about the fact that both papers refer to the same study by including a clear **trial identifier**.

If you are preparing a plan for multiple publications the key messages for each publication should be clearly stated. If you are a professional writer being briefed about a study, remember that a key message needs a verb and be prepared to challenge vague statements such as 'this paper is about the efficacy of Wunderdrug'.

If there is no chance of all authors discussing a publication face to face, circulating an **outline** can be a good way to generate discussion (and, with luck, agreement) on the key message(s).

■ Key people / players

The really important people in developing any publication are its authors. Make sure you have included everybody who qualifies (and read the section on **authorship** if you are in doubt). Remember, too, that other people such as your boss, or representatives from the funding organisation, may need to be involved. Allow sufficient time for everybody to comment on planned publications and try to work out the most efficient way of gathering comments and deciding who sees what, and when.

While all authors should have ample opportunity to contribute to a publication it may also help to identify 'key people' among the authors. Ideally, the entire writing group will meet to discuss the planned publication at various stages, for example developing the outline and agreeing the final version. However, it is sometimes impossible for everyone to meet face to face, and telephone conferences with more than five people can be frustrating and unproductive. In such cases, there may be a temptation to work more closely with one or two of the authors, and have slightly less contact with the others. This pattern is rarely a strategic decision, but sometimes arises because of difficulties of working across different time zones.

Working with an 'inner' and 'outer' writing group can cause problems and delays if the 'inner' group does not include everybody with strong views about the publication. If the 'inner' group takes decisions without consulting the others, this is unlikely to lead to good relations, and may even cause delays if the authors who were not consulted insist on major changes at a late stage. Try to avoid this situation by making sure everybody comments on the outline, so there are no surprises when a draft is produced.

■ Key words

Many journals ask authors to identify a few key words. These are designed to help the indexing services (such as **Medline**) classify papers correctly. Check the 'Instructions to authors' guidance notes for specific requirements but, in the absence of these, consider using the Medical Subject Headings (MeSH) used by Medline.

Unless you are very familiar with **MeSH headings** check before you select, to make sure you have got them right.

You can check MeSH headings at www.nlm.nih.gov/mesh/.

L

■ Last author

See **order of authors** for a full discussion of this subject. In many disciplines the position of last author is endowed with special status and may be competed over almost as fiercely as the first. However, this status has never been defined, and the convention appears to vary between countries and specialties. Although the

International Committee of Medical Journal Editors (ICMJE) (Vancouver) criteria clearly state that obtaining funding or overall supervision of a department does not, alone, merit authorship, the last place has often been reserved for just such a person. *See* **guest authors** for more details. The trend for journals to list individuals' contributions rather than just their names and titles may reduce the prevalence of undeserving guest authors, but it is too early to tell whether it will abolish the jostling for last place.

In some cases, the **corresponding author** or **guarantor** occupies the last position but, again, there is no rule about this. While authors often claim to know what is so special about being last on the list, readers may, of course, be happily ignorant of this convention, or may apply the traditions of their own specialty, which may be different from those of the authors. The only rule in deciding who goes last (or first) is to discover all authors' understandings and expectations and to try to agree this as amicably as possible.

Marušić A, Hren D, Mansi B *et al.* (2014) Five-step authorship framework to improve transparency in disclosing contributions to industry-sponsored clinical trial publications. *BMC Med.* **12**: 197.

■ Late breaker abstracts

Submission deadlines are sometimes so long in advance of major conferences that there is a danger that only rather old research gets presented. Some meetings therefore allow 'late breaker abstracts' for new findings. You may have to provide evidence that your data were not available by the regular submission deadline, you are likely to be restricted to a **poster presentation**, rather than an **oral** one, and your **abstract** may not appear in the conference book, or may appear in a separate section, but it is worth enquiring if your target meeting permits late breakers if you have a genuine problem in hitting the regular submission deadline.

■ Lead time

(Pronounced like a dog leash, not like the heavy element.)

This is the time between acceptance and publication. Lead times used to be substantial in the days of print journals when editors had strict page budgets but often accepted more submissions than they had space for, which then waited in a queue, often for months, until space was available in the print journal. Lead time may still be an important factor in your choice of journal if it is important to have copies of your article by a certain date (e.g. for a big conference). However, since most journals now publish articles on their website as soon as they are ready, and since accepted articles may be cited as being 'in press', you will probably be more concerned about the **decision time** than the lead time.

Some journals publish the acceptance date at the bottom of an article – in this case you can easily work out the average lead time. If this information is not available and you need to discover it, you should consult the website or contact the editorial office.

Most journals publish accepted articles on their websites before they appear in print. Such articles are listed as '**epub** ahead of print' on Medline. Electronic posting of the final version is considered to be publication and in some journals the electronic rather than the print version is now considered the definitive one. However, if you want **offprints** you will also need to know when the printed version will appear. Articles can be cited with a permanent (and useful) reference even before they have been assigned volume or page numbers thanks to the **DOI system**.

See Chapter 3 'How long will it take?' (pp. 13–17) for more details.

■ Legends; *see* figure legends

■ Letters to the editor

■ Writing

Journals publish two distinct types of letters: those that comment on published material, and those that contain new research findings. Some indexing systems treat these differently (usually including the latter but ignoring the former). You should therefore check the journal (and, if necessary, the indexing system) before considering using a letter to present new findings. Research letters may be a useful format for studies with straightforward methods that can be compressed into a strict word limit. The acceptance rate and speed of publication for research letters are often slightly more favourable than those for full articles.

The more traditional correspondence column can be useful to draw attention to your own publications or to offer supplementary information pertinent to the point being discussed. However, most journals accept letters only if they relate to something the journal has published. Some also set a time limit for receiving such letters (e.g. 3 weeks after the original publication in *NEJM*) which means you need to keep up to date with the literature, and be prepared to respond quickly.

■ Responding

If your publication stimulates letters that the journal plans to publish you will normally be given the opportunity to respond. If they receive several letters, print journals usually try to publish them together, along with the author's response. Production schedules mean that this correspondence often appears several months after the original publication (at least for print journals), but the journal may not give you much time to prepare a response, since letters are usually slotted into issues after other sections, so the decision to publish them is usually taken shortly before publication. This also means that you may not see a proof of your response, or may receive only a **galley** (not a **page**) **proof**.

In contrast, a few journals (notably *The BMJ* and *PLOS One*) use their websites to encourage rapid, electronic responses. Authors may choose to respond to each letter individually or even enter into a dialogue with the responder. The corresponding author will usually be alerted when responses are posted – and it is a nice idea to let other authors know.

Try to address the points made by correspondents as succinctly and politely as possible (journal editors do not want letters that are long or defamatory) and consult your co-authors before you reply. It may help to treat the letters in the same way that you would approach reviewers' comments. In other words, take a deep breath, calm down, and try to be as objective as possible. Nobody likes having their interpretation called into question or flaws in their research brought to light, but remember that this is the way that science is meant to proceed, and at least the letter proves that somebody has read your paper and considers your work sufficiently interesting to comment on it.

Peter Gøtzsche and colleagues did an interesting study of author responses to criticism in *The BMJ*'s Rapid Responses. They found that only about half of the authors responded to substantive criticisms of their publication and therefore suggested that editors should do more to ensure a better response.

Gøtzsche PC, Delamothe T, Godlee F *et al.* (2010) Adequacy of authors' replies to criticism raised in electronic letters to the editor: cohort study. *BMJ.* **341**: c3926.

M

■ Masked review; *see* blinded review

■ Meat extenders

A term coined by Ed Huth (former editor of *Annals of Internal Medicine*) to describe the act of 'blending data from one study with additional data to extract yet another paper that could not make its way on the second set of data alone'.[1] Thus, a form of **redundant publication**. But it raises the question of why this form of malpractice inspired such meaty metaphors (*see* **salami science**).

1 Huth E (1986) Irresponsible authorship and wasteful publication. *Ann Intern Med.* **104**: 257–9.

■ Media relations

A good publication strategy, especially one for a commercial product or major research project, should be accompanied by a broader communication strategy covering plans for working with the press (newspapers, television, radio, etc.). Except in the smallest of organisations, the nerdy scientific stuff (i.e. journal articles) and trendy media bits (i.e. public relations or PR) are usually handled by different people, with different hairstyles and pay packages, but it makes sense if these two worlds communicate. In particular, publication planners need to make sure that the PR folk don't get over-enthusiastic and issue **press releases** before publication which might seriously mess up your chances of getting into a good journal. However, people involved with publications should share their plans so that the PR people can do their job and seize appropriate opportunities for corporate trumpet-blowing. Many of the major journals and publishers have their own press departments who are happy to cooperate over issuing press releases and editors are delighted when their publications get picked up by the general media.

Journalistic interest in presentations at meetings is less straightforward, especially if your results have been submitted to or accepted by, but not yet published in, a major journal. Check the journal's press **embargo** policies carefully and make sure you do not fall foul of them. Some journals even expect you to withdraw presentations from conferences once they have accepted your paper – but others are more relaxed about this. Just occasionally, you may be able to orchestrate the perfect combination of a presentation at a big conference occurring simultaneously (or just hours before) publication in a prestigious journal with joint press activities. Such impressive choreography requires exciting results, a cooperative journal and a fair bit of luck with your timing.

Editors accept that journalists may attend scientific meetings and report the most interesting findings. However, they do not welcome authors (or their institutions or companies) actively seeking press coverage by holding **press conferences** or issuing press releases before a full paper is published. Since abstracts are considered to be in the public domain, it is acceptable to give these to journalists who request information but providing slides or copies of posters is risky as it could lead to extensive coverage that a journal would consider to be **prior publication**.

■ Medical writers

See Chapter 4 'Working with a medical writer' (pp. 19–21).

If a professional writer works on a manuscript, their involvement, and more importantly who paid for it, should always be acknowledged. Most journals follow the **International Committee of Medical Journal Editors' (ICMJE)** criteria for authorship and do not consider a writer who has not been involved in the design or conduct of the study as an author. However, one or two journals interpret the criteria differently and feel that anybody who helps write a manuscript must be an author (*see* **acknowledgements** for details). Professional writers whose contribution is properly acknowledged (either in the acknowledgements, as contributors or even as authors) are not **ghost writers** (because they are visible). However, this rather insulting term is often used and sometimes gets confused with **ghost authors**, which constitute a quite different spooky problem.

■ Medline

A bibliographic database, run by the US National Library of Medicine, covering around 5000 medical journals with entries from 1949. Medline is probably the most widely used, although not the most comprehensive, database for doctors searching the literature since it is available free on the internet via **PubMed** (www. ncbi.nlm.nih.gov/PubMed). For this reason, articles in journals that are included in Medline are more likely to be retrieved (or at least their abstracts read) by researchers than those that are not listed, so inclusion in Medline is an important consideration when choosing a **target journal**.

Medline includes the title and author details and usually an abstract, but never the full text of an article. However, full text of some articles is now available on **PubMed Central** which can be searched from the same website.

■ Meeting choice; *see* congress / conference choice

■ Meetings (of the writing group)

The fastest, most efficient and probably most pleasant way to discuss and get agreement on publication strategy is for the **writing group** to meet. If your budget and diaries permit, try to organise at least two meetings. The first should be held as soon as results are available. The purpose of this meeting is to agree the **key message(s)**, confirm the membership of the writing group and their tasks, and thus finalise the authors for each publication. Ideally, you should already have some idea of how many abstracts or papers you plan to publish and who they are aimed at. Now that you know the results you can firm up these plans and select your target and second-choice journals and target conference(s). The decisions taken at this meeting will form the core of your publication strategy. Appoint somebody to take and circulate notes of decisions made and action points. Once the strategy is agreed, you should produce a detailed plan showing target dates for milestones such as first draft, review, submission, etc. *See* Chapter 3 'How long will it take?' (pp. 13–17) and Chapter 2 'Developing a publication plan for a multicentre study' (pp. 7–11) for more details.

The second meeting should take place when you have a reasonably mature draft and all **key players** have had a chance to contribute. The object of this meeting is to agree a final version for submission. Setting a date for the second meeting is harder than for the first, since there is little point in meeting if your paper still requires a lot of detailed work but you risk delaying submission if you wait too long. You should therefore schedule two or three possible dates at the first meeting and try to persuade members to keep them free.

If members of the writing group and all other key players can agree on the final wording of the submission by e-mail, you may not need a second meeting. However, if there are differences of opinion, a meeting is usually the swiftest way to resolve them. If a meeting is impossible, a telephone (or video) conference is the next best thing, and definitely preferable to endless rounds of e-mail. Once again, appoint somebody to record decisions and circulate notes to all attendees and to any key players who could not take part.

■ Mega-journal

This term is used, sometimes rather loosely, to describe journals that use peer review only to check that the research is sound and clearly reported rather than to judge whether articles are likely to be of interest to readers. The most obvious example of a mega-journal is *PLOS One*, which definitely deserves the name as it publishes more articles per year than any other journal. However, the term is also used to describe much smaller journals which use similar selection criteria (making pedants like me gnash their teeth and write blogs suggesting more accurate names).[1] As with any type of journal, the desirability of mega-journals as targets for your work depends on what you are looking for. If you want a high chance of acceptance, they are good news; if you yearn to be published somewhere exclusive and prestigious, they are a disaster. Mega-journals tend to offer (or at least advertise) relatively rapid and straightforward publication, but the reputable ones are properly peer reviewed so this process inevitably takes a while as it relies on unpaid reviewers and often, also, unpaid academic editors. Given the unselective nature of mega-journals, it is perhaps inevitable that their **impact factors** are on the low side, but paradoxically, they may compare favourably with some specialty journals with much higher rejection rates. For example, *PLOS One*'s 2014 impact factor is 3.23 while the *European Journal of Anaesthesiology*'s is 2.94. As ever with **journal choice**, it is important to discover all the authors' **expectations** (and their prejudices), agree some criteria, research potential journals carefully and then try to reach an amicable decision.

1 Wager E (2011) Journals that dare not speak their name. *The BMJ* blogs. http://blogs. bmj.com/bmj/2011/03/22.

■ MeSH headings

A system of Medical Subject Headings used to categorise entries by the US National Library of Medicine's **Medline** and used by some journals for key words. The full list can be found at www.ncbi.nlm.nih.gov/mesh. (Incidentally, this website provides a nice example of bureaucrats' love of long words, as it describes the self-explanatory 'medical subject headings' as 'the NLM controlled vocabulary thesaurus'.) Even if a journal does not specify that you should use MeSH headings for key words they are a good starting point and may help ensure your publication is correctly coded if it is listed on Medline.

■ Metrics

Cynics, according to Oscar Wilde, are people who know 'the price of everything and the value of nothing'. Sadly, this description applies to many bosses who don't understand the importance of publications. Even if you are lucky enough to work for a more enlightened manager, you are likely to have to justify your budget or your fees at some point, so you may need to resort to metrics (which is just a fancy term for measuring what you do).

However, unlike many other industrial processes, where it is relatively easy to demonstrate efficiencies and to prove the value of what you do, it is remarkably tricky to devise sensible metrics for publication activities. For example, if you measured the success of a team by how often they got papers accepted in their first target journal, this would probably ensure that they never submitted anything to the top journals with the lowest acceptance rates but the highest impact factors. Conversely, if you rate publications only by the impact factor of the journal in which they are published, this could encourage time-wasting strategies with unrealistic target journals.

Another problem in publication metrics is that it often makes good sense to hold back some publications while speeding up others. For instance, you should not publish secondary papers before primary ones, so setting fixed targets for all papers (e.g. aiming to submit all papers within 4 months of results becoming available) doesn't make sense. It also seems unfair to hold authors, writers or planners entirely responsible for delays caused by journals' peer-review or production processes – although perhaps they should take some responsibility for choosing a slow journal in the first place.

Discussing metrics with people from other companies, for example at **ISMPP** meetings, may offer helpful insights, but don't expect companies to share all their performance secrets willingly. If your company takes part in 'benchmarking' (i.e. sharing data with a group of companies usually via a consultant to establish industry norms and identify best practice) you might be able to get information about how long companies take to publish their clinical trials, on average.

If you are an in-house publication team and need to justify your budget you can ask a couple of friendly agencies about their standard fees for producing various types of publication and use this to demonstrate your productivity. But trying to show that your publications are better than others, or that your publication strategy is top notch, is always going to involve some subjective judgements, so don't expect this to be an easy or uncontroversial process. If you get into unproductive arguments, try using the quote at the beginning of this section.

N

■ Names

Think about how the authors' names will appear in the journal, in references, and in indexes such as **Medline**. If you use the format 'full given name, surname' (e.g. John Smith) this will appear as Smith, J in indexes and there will be no information about middle names. If you use the format 'initials, surname' (i.e. J E Smith) or 'first name, initials, surname' (i.e. John E Smith), the name will appear as Smith, J E in indexes and reference lists. It is up to the author to indicate how his or her name should appear, but most people prefer to use their full names, especially if short versions start with a different letter (e.g. my friends call me Liz, but I use Elizabeth for publications).

Take particular care with multi-part names or those in which the family name appears before the individual name. English language journals and bibliographic systems are often embarrassingly poor at handling Spanish or Chinese names.

Accents on names often disappear when you submit abstracts or papers electronically. There is not much you can do about abstracts, as you rarely see proofs, although you could try e-mailing the conference organisers; but for papers, check proofs carefully for any non-standard characters (such as the Croatian diacritics I love so much!). However, incorrect indexing of names may be a thing of the past, thanks to the **ORCID** system which provides a unique research identifier.

Indexing systems sometimes garble, or ignore, group names.[1] This is a shame, as it may discourage their use. To increase the chances of your paper being retrieved correctly, it is safest to include individual members of the **writing group** as well as a group name (e.g. M Barassment & N Continent on behalf of the DRIBBLE study group). Journals that list people's contributions and include a study **guarantor** always require individuals to be listed in addition to a study group.

See also **order of authors**, **group authorship**.

1 Dickersin K, Scherer R, Suci ES *et al.* (2002) Problems with indexing and citation of articles with group authorship. *JAMA*. **287**: 2772–4.

■ Negative studies

Studies may be termed 'negative' if they produce statistically non-significant differences between groups, or if they produce results that are disappointing or inconvenient for the sponsor or authors. In the past, many negative studies (of both varieties) were never published, leading to considerable problems with **publication bias**. The lack of publication was partly due to the difficulty of getting such studies accepted (especially those that failed to reach statistical significance and thus produced inconclusive results) but much more often was due to them never being submitted for publication. One reason why many journals require **trial registration** is to reduce the problem of non-publication, or at least make it visible. The advent of less selective, electronic journals such as *PLOS One*, which have a policy of publishing all sound science regardless of the direction of the results, has largely overcome the problem of finding a home for such reports; in fact, there are now even journals that specialise in negative studies. The Medical Publishing Insights and Practices Initiative provides a list of such journals: www. mpip-initiative.org/news/12/61/List-of-Journals.

Since 2008, the Declaration of Helsinki has stated that doctors have a duty to publish all studies regardless of whether they produce positive or negative results. **Good Publication Practice (GPP3)** states that 'results should be submitted for publication in a peer-reviewed journal regardless of whether the findings are positive, negative, or inconclusive or whether the studied intervention is investigational, is licensed, or has been discontinued or withdrawn from the market'. Publication policies should enforce this principle.

■ Nitpickers

Every place of work has somebody who can spot a typo at a hundred paces and delights in a misplaced apostrophe. If you handle them carefully you can use such nitpickers to your advantage. The following rules will help:

- never show your first draft to a nitpicker
- if possible, wait until several other people have reviewed a manuscript before you ask a nitpicker to read it
- as with other reviewers, give the nitpicker clear information about the status of the manuscript, which parts cannot be changed, exactly what you would like him/her to do and by when.

Used this way, a keen-eyed reviewer, or somebody with a good sense of grammar and style, can be an ally. Nitpickers should not be confused with **vicious reviewers** who make personal attacks and take pleasure in tearing apart other researchers' work. Although nitpickers can be annoying, remember that a really thorough **internal review** is usually less painful than a dressing down from the journal's reviewers and it may increase your chances of acceptance. Even though good science should shine through a poorly prepared manuscript, appearances do matter, and a polished paper is likely to impress reviewers and editors. *See* **proofs (page proofs)** – when nitpickers can be really useful.

■ Number of authors

The number of authors on each publication should be determined by established criteria. *See* **authorship** for more details. Whatever criteria are used, they must be applied equally to everybody involved with the study. Some sponsor companies, aware that readers' and reviewers' perceptions might be affected by seeing several employees on the author list, try to play down their involvement and may try to restrict the number of employee authors (or even forbid them altogether) creating **ghost authors**. It is up to the other authors to explain that this is unacceptable. The move from a simple **by-line** to the **contributorship** system may discourage this practice, since it may be apparent that a **key person** (e.g. a statistician) has been omitted.

The **International Committee of Medical Journal Editors' (ICMJE)** Recommendations state that contributors who do not meet the authorship criteria should not be listed, and that all those who do meet the criteria should be included. The 2013 revision of the ICMJE Recommendations also states that all authors should be prepared to take accountability for the work. **Good Publication Practice (GPP)** also encourages companies to apply criteria consistently to employees and external investigators.

Since all authors must contribute to the publication, in addition to their contribution to the research itself, establishing a **writing group** can help to distinguish those who qualify for authorship from other investigators (who may be listed as **collaborators**).

Large studies may have many authors. However, as a general rule, the more authors there are, the longer a publication will take to develop. For short reports or case studies an interminable list of authors may stretch the credibility of readers and reviewers and raise suspicions of **guest authorship**.

Although it is rarely spelled out in conference guidelines, the same authorship conventions apply for abstracts as for full papers. However, local investigators may sometimes be added to the author list if they are presenting findings at a local meeting.

■ Number of publications

Deciding how many publications you can squeeze out of your research is one of the most important strategic decisions you will have to make. Sadly, there is no simple formula to guide you. The findings of some enormous and important studies can be neatly summed up in a single paper, while other studies may warrant all sorts of secondary publications. For academics seeking to enrich their CVs, or companies hoping to promote their product, it may be tempting to try to produce masses of publications but if you overstep the limits of reasonableness you may stand accused of **salami science** or **redundant publication**. However tempting it may be to dream of dozens of publications, try to keep readers and editors in mind and think about what they want. It can be frustrating to have to piece together several bits of jigsaw that should really have been published as a whole. Also, if your strategy produces many overlapping papers, you may find that editors do not want to publish them, so you would have been better off with more modest ambitions and fewer, meatier, publications.

O

■ Offprints

These are individual copies of a paper ordered before publication (as opposed to **reprints** which, strictly speaking, are printed separately, after the original version has been published; however, the terms are sometimes used interchangeably). Because they are printed at the same time as the complete journal, offprints are usually cheaper than reprints ordered after publication. Offprint order forms are usually sent with the proofs and must be returned quickly. You should therefore establish how many offprints are needed (by consulting all authors, the sponsor and anybody else likely to want copies) as soon as the paper is accepted. Do not wait to work out how many offprints you need until the proofs arrive – large companies often take several weeks to sort out purchase orders or check how many copies their affiliate companies want and this could delay the proofs and therefore publication. Since the price of offprints usually depends on the length of the article you may not get an exact figure until page proofs are produced. However, you can get a price chart from the publisher and ask the editor in charge of production for an estimate of how many pages your article will fill.

Open Access journals may permit or even encourage you or your company to print your own copies or to send electronic offprints (e.g. PDF files) but check with the journal before assuming that this is allowed as some licences do not permit commercial reuse. (*See* **Creative Commons licences** for more details.)

■ Ombudsman / ombudsperson

One or two journals have appointed ombudsmen to hear grievances from disgruntled authors or readers. These ombudsmen are usually respected academics who are independent from the journal. Their role is to adjudicate in disagreements that cannot be settled satisfactorily by the editorial team. *See* **appeals** for more details.

Warlow C (2011) Ombudsman's ninth report. *Lancet*. **378**: 548–9.

Horton R (1998) The journal ombudsperson: a step toward scientific press oversight. *JAMA*. **280**: 298–9.

Both references describe *The Lancet*'s system.

■ Open Access journals

Journals can be categorised according to who pays for access to their contents. In the traditional funding model, journals make their full contents available only to those who have paid a subscription to the print or electronic versions, or those who pay for access to a particular item (sometimes called 'pay-per-view'). In contrast, Open Access journals are freely available, on the web, to all readers, and authors usually pay an **article processing charge**.

According to the 'Berlin declaration',[1] Open Access journals must allow authors to retain copyright on their work and must deposit their contents in a permanent repository (e.g. **PubMed Central**) to ensure it doesn't disappear. Journals that meet these requirements usually refer to themselves as Open Access (with capital O and A) to distinguish themselves from other publications that may be freely available on the web but don't meet the other Berlin criteria.

The trend towards Open Access gathered momentum in the late 1990s with the expansion of electronic publishing. Open Access has some influential supporters especially among academic institutions who find it increasingly hard to pay hefty journal subscription rates. Some large research sponsors (notably the US National Institutes of Health, Wellcome Trust and UK Medical Research Council) now require their studies to be published in Open Access journals. As a result, some commercial publishers have agreed to a compromise position of making all or part of their publications available some time after the initial publication. For example, you can access research papers (but not commentaries) from *JAMA* and the *New England Journal of Medicine* on their journal websites 6 months after they appear in the paper journal. Other publishers have responded by offering Open Access as an option to authors for a fee (usually between $1000 and $5000 per article; see, for example, www.oxfordjournals.org/oxfordopen/). Other publishers do not provide access from their own websites but allow authors to deposit copies in an institutional repository (this is often referred to as **Green Open Access**).

When selecting a journal you should consider how accessible it is, especially if you want your work to be read beyond academic institutions or in resource-poor countries. The **Open Access Scholarly Publishers Association (OASPA)** and **Directory of Open Access Journals (DOAJ)** provide useful lists of Open Access journals.

1 Berlin declaration (2003). www.oa.mpg.de/openaccess-berlin/berlindeclaration.html

Tamber PS, Godlee F and Newmark P (2003) Open access to peer-reviewed research: making it happen. *Lancet*. **362**: 1575–7.

■ Open Access Scholarly Publishers Association (OASPA)

OASPA is a trade organisation which was established in 2008 and represents, as its name suggests, many Open Access publishers. It also includes several traditional publishers such as Wiley and Springer which publish both subscription and Open Access journals. It requires members to follow a code of conduct and was involved in developing the 'Principles of transparency and best practice in scholarly publishing' jointly with the **Directory of Open Access Journals (DOAJ)** and the **Committee on Publication Ethics (COPE)**.

http://oaspa.org/

DOAJ (2014) Principles of transparency and best practice in scholarly publishing. https://doaj.org/bestpractice

■ OpenDOAR (the Directory of Open Access Repositories)

A handy tool to identify institutional repositories (it lists nearly 3000 of them from all around the world).

www.opendoar.org/

■ Open peer review

A review in which the reviewer's identity is revealed to the author(s). *See* **blinded (masked) review** and **review process** for details of other systems.

■ Oral presentations

Talks given at conferences are called oral presentations (following the curious scientific tradition of preferring long words to short ones). Since time is more limited than space most meetings accept relatively few submissions for oral presentations and the bulk are presented as posters. Talks are therefore considered more prestigious than posters and are more likely to generate media attention. However, some conferences allow authors to indicate their preference for an oral or poster presentation. Consider opting for a poster if the person who will present the research does not speak the language used at the meeting fluently: remember that, as well as delivering the talk, the presenter will have to answer questions, and cannot always follow a script.

Good preparation is the key to a good talk and also permits co-authors to comment. Treat the slides like any other publication and make sure you get input from all **key players**. The presentation should be a team effort not an opportunity for the presenter to air his or her personal theories or pet interests. *See* **slides** for more details.

To avoid jeopardising the full publication, you should not distribute copies of your slides to journalists, although you may provide your abstract and answer their questions. Perhaps surprisingly, most journals do not consider a 'webcast' from a meeting to constitute **prior publication**.[1]

The key to obtaining an oral presentation is to craft a persuasive **abstract** but it is not always easy to convey your findings in a few words. Having a clear message and identifying the interests and needs of your audience are important factors for success. Having interesting results also helps.

1 Kassirer JP (1999) Posting presentations at medical meetings on the internet. *N Engl J Med.* **340**: 803.

■ ORCID (Open Researcher and Contributor ID)

Names are useful for identifying authors and their publications when they are relatively unusual (like Elizabeth Wager) but almost useless if you are trying to work out what J Smith or K Lee has published. This can be important if you want to check somebody's publication record, claim publications as your own or inspect earlier publications of a researcher who has committed misconduct. The ORCID system (http://orcid.org/) allocates individual researchers a unique identifier and journals are increasingly using this, so you may need it for submission. The system has the advantage that, in future, it should be easier to track down authors (or potential peer reviewers) even if they have changed institutions and e-mails, assuming they keep their central ORCID record up to date.

It's free to register for an ORCID identifier and I can't think of any good reason why authors don't do so. I've even blogged about it.

http://blogs.bmj.com/bmj/2012/08/01/liz-wager-an-orcid-by-any-other-name-would-smell-as-sweet/

■ Order of authors

This can cause all sorts of problems and neither individual journals nor the **International Committee of Medical Journal Editors (ICMJE)** gives any advice on the subject. The main problem is that everybody thinks they know what the listing order implies but, in fact, conventions vary between disciplines and between countries.

Perhaps the only firm fact is that most people regard the first named author as the most important. The author/date (Harvard) reference system emphasises this by identifying publications by their first author in the text (e.g. Wager *et al.*, 2003).

The last position on the **by-line** sometimes indicates seniority or overall supervision. However, this is not universally true. *See* **number of authors** and **guest authors** if you are tempted to add a prestigious 'guest' to your author list.

Various systems have been devised for more democratic or transparent listing but, since you normally cannot explain what system you have used, readers are usually none the wiser. Listing by alphabetical order may seem fair if your name is Dr Aaronson, but will probably be less attractive to Dr Zblinski (or even Dr Wager).

Some researchers have proposed mathematical formulae to determine author order.[1] However, these have not been widely adopted and are unlikely to solve your problems, since they rely on subjective assessments about who did what, and what each contribution is worth – which is usually what authorship disagreements are about.

The most practical advice is to discuss the order of authors as soon as you have agreed who will be listed. Discover the expectations and perceptions of all co-authors/contributors and try to reach an amicable agreement. Do *not* leave this to the final draft or just before the deadline for submission.

If a study will generate several publications you may be able to placate disgruntled co-authors by using different orders for each paper.

1 Hunt R (1991) Trying an authorship index. *Nature.* **352**: 187.

Bhopal RS, Rankin JM, McColl E *et al.* (1997) The vexed question of authorship: views of researchers in a British medical faculty. *BMJ.* **314**: 1009–12.

Bhopal RS, Rankin JM, McColl E *et al.* (1997) Authorship. Team approach to assigning authorship order is recommended. *BMJ.* **314**: 1046.

■ Organisations

Some journals retain close links with their parent organisation (usually an academic society). This may mean that they give priority to material presented at the society's meetings or from its members. Check these links when choosing your **target journal** to see if they could work for or against you.

Some meetings restrict abstract submission to members of the organising society, or require that a member sponsors every abstract. Check these requirements well before the submission deadline to prevent delays.

■ Outlines

Although you may be keen to rush into the first draft, preparing an outline of a planned publication is time well spent. The main advantage of an outline is that it allows you to decide on the contents of the paper and to get agreement from all **key players** before you commit time and effort to preparing a full draft. It is far better to discover differences in interpretation at this stage than after you have spent days writing a draft. The outline also bridges the gap between agreeing the **key messages**, which are, by definition, simplified and concise, and elaborating on these. An outline can also prevent overlaps or omissions and improve consistency when several people are writing a paper or when several papers are planned from a single study.

Even if you have circulated notes about the publication strategy it is a good idea to restate the main decisions (e.g. target audience, target journal and second-choice journal) on the outline. You should also indicate important target journal requirements such as word limits and special formatting instructions, e.g. Abstract (structured, maximum 250 words).

All key players should review the outline, not just the authors. For some reason, people often pay less attention to reviewing an outline than to reviewing a full draft. You may therefore need to explain why you are circulating an outline and to remind key players that publication may be delayed if they raise major queries about the structure of the paper or the **key message(s)** after this stage.

■ Overlapping publications; *see* redundant publication

■ Ownership of data

This can be a thorny issue and it is therefore important that ownership is clearly set out in the **investigators' agreement** or **publication agreement**. Ownership of data should not be confused with **access to data**. Many research sponsors assert that data from a trial that they have funded belongs to them; even if this is the case, there should be a clause in the agreement that investigators will have access to the data and will be free to publish. The term 'data' can also have varying interpretations. It is a condition of most research that individual (unanonymised) patient data remain confidential and are not shared. The only exceptions are accounts of serious adverse events which may, of necessity, contain information by which a patient could be identified. In practice, access to data usually therefore means access to the analysed (not raw) dataset or to anonymised patient-level data.

Problems can arise if investigators want to perform additional (i.e. secondary) analyses. Ideally, all statistical analyses are agreed beforehand and set out in the **data analysis plan**. The sponsor and investigators should therefore discuss this and agree what analyses will (and will not) be done. If the results reveal unexpected findings it may be acceptable to do some secondary, explorative analyses. **Good Publication Practice** (GPP3) states that study sponsors should 'provide reasonable additional analyses' in support of publications, if the authors request them. However, investigators must realise that sponsors do not have unlimited time or budgets for these. It is also important to get statistical advice about whether such analyses are meaningful. Too many analyses could constitute '**data dredging**'.

If you are employed at an academic institution you should check your employment contract as well as individual funding agreements, especially if you may move and hope to be able to take data with you. In most cases, contracts stipulate that the data belong to the institution (which may come as a surprise to you) so always check the small print. Government employees and contractors should not expect to own any data they produce (and therefore are not usually able to assign copyright to a journal, since it is not theirs to give away), so check before you make any assumptions.

P

■ Page budget

Most printed journals that use a subscription funding model run to a page budget; in other words, the editor knows that each issue or volume of the journal must not exceed a certain length agreed with the publisher. This makes economic sense if printing and distribution are a major cost (which they are for traditional printed journals) and if the journal's income is largely derived from subscriptions that are paid in advance each year (so there is no way to go back to readers and ask for more money once it has been spent). However, page budgets can cause a lengthy **lead time** if editors accept more papers than they can publish each year. **Electronic publishing** has changed all this. Purely electronic journals have no limit on space and therefore no need for a queue of papers. Even journals that retain a print version may alleviate the problem of long lead times by making accepted papers available on their website before they appear in print. Journals may also keep print costs down by following the 'Electronic long, paper short' (**ELPS**) system.

■ Page charges; *see* article processing charge (APC)

■ *PeerJ*

This **Open Access** journal has some innovative features, including a novel author payment model, relaxed **formatting requirements** and a **preprint** function. Instead of the journal demanding an **article processing charge**, each author must pay a subscription fee that allows them to publish a certain number of articles per year, for life. Author subscriptions in 2015 were $99 for one and $199 for two articles per year. Therefore, for articles with fewer than 10 authors, the cost of publication in *PeerJ* is considerably lower than for many other Open Access journals. *PeerJ* covers biology and medicine.

https://peerj.com/

■ Peers

It has been claimed, probably by somebody who just received a crushing rejection, that the truly original have no peers, but, for the rest of us, submissions are judged by reviewers whom journal editors consider our equals, or at least up to the job. Several authors have been unable to resist puns about peering into peer review, although, so far as I know, none has drawn analogies to the ermine-clad members of the UK House of Lords (and I am still unsure why they are called peers since they would seem to be definitely more equal than others).

Some journals ask authors to suggest people who might review their paper. This is even a requirement for electronic submission to some journals, and, if this is the case, you should agree some suitable names with your co-authors before you submit. You should not propose anybody who has been involved with the research being reported, nor anybody working at the same institution as the author(s). Some journals will follow authors' suggestions in most cases, while others chiefly use such information to enlarge their reviewer database. Unless your target journal practises **open peer review** you will probably never know if your suggestions have been followed.

Even when editors use a reviewer suggested by the author, they will almost certainly also approach at least one other reviewer from the journal's database. Although authors expect to be judged by their peers (i.e. people of similar standing), it has been known for senior researchers to delegate the job of reviewing to their juniors and they do not always inform the journal about this. While journal editors and authors might feel aggrieved about this (if they are aware of it), there is evidence[1] that younger scientists actually produce more conscientious and helpful reviews than older ones, so such delegation may not be entirely a bad thing (although it would be better if people were honest about it).

If you feel that a reviewer has misunderstood your research, it might be worth writing an **appeal** to the editor, especially if another reviewer has recognised the merits of your paper. However, be careful to be as objective as possible, and avoid attacking the reviewer's education or intelligence (whether you know their identity or not). If the review was anonymous do not suggest that you know the reviewer's identity. For one thing, it undermines the principles of anonymous review and may make the editor uneasy, and for another, you might be wrong.

1 Black N, van Rooyen S, Godlee F *et al.* (1998) What makes a good reviewer and a good review for a general medical journal? *JAMA.* **280**: 231–3.

■ Permissions

You need the copyright holder's permission to reproduce a figure, table or substantial chunk of text in a publication. Copyright law is rather vague about what constitutes a substantial amount of text but the UK Society of Authors advises that quotations of fewer than 400 words do not require permission. Remember that the author is not necessarily the copyright holder, so even if you wrote the original publication you may still need to get permission from the publisher. Ownership of copyright depends on the source. As a general rule, for subscription-based journals and for books, it tends to be the publisher. But **Open Access journals** usually have different arrangements under which the authors retain copyright (*see* **Creative Commons licences**).

Allow plenty of time to sort out permissions. Some publishers respond rapidly (Elsevier takes 10 days), but some can take weeks or even months (e.g. the *Journal of Clinical Oncology* takes up to 30 working days). You will also need to think about your budget. Some publishers demand payment but fees vary depending on the planned use and could be substantial for commercial material, electronic distribution or commercial meetings. Publishers generally do not charge individual authors for republication in an academic journal or presentation at a scientific conference but may charge commercial companies for this.

You can usually find details about obtaining permission on the journal or publisher's website. In other cases, send your request to the publisher (not to the academic editor).

Although you should apply for permission as soon as possible, you cannot do this before you have selected your **target journal** or meeting, or have a rough idea of when the paper might be published, or the presentation given, since most publishers request this information. You will also need precise details of what you hope to reproduce (e.g. the figure or table and page number, plus the full reference). Check that the item has not been taken from another publication (e.g. read the legend for any acknowledgements) and, if it has, track down the primary source and approach the original copyright holder, since the intermediate owner (i.e. the second journal or book publisher) will not be able to grant you permission.

Keep a copy of permission letters since some journals require these before they will publish your paper. You should also note any requirements for the way in which the permission is acknowledged.

■ Personal communications

If you want to quote something that somebody has said but not formally published you will probably need to resort to a 'personal communication'. First, check the instructions of your target journal to see if this kind of attribution is acceptable (some journals do not allow them).

Unlike reference citations, which usually give only the author's family name (e.g. Smith, 1999), personal communications usually indicate the first name (presumably to avoid misattribution to other people with the same surname). For example 'Up to 60% of people who attend publishing workshops fall asleep after lunch (personal communication: Dr Elizabeth Wager)'.

Some journals require even fuller details, for example *Circulation* demands details of the originating person's qualifications, *Blood* requires the person's affiliation, *JAMA* requires the date and the method of communication (oral or written). Some journals (e.g. *JAMA* and the *Journal of Antimicrobial Chemotherapy*) require signed permission from anybody who is mentioned in this way. In any case, it is courteous to check with the person you wish to name, and they might even be able to provide a 'proper' reference if they have subsequently published their observation. If your target journal requires written evidence, or details such as the qualifications and affiliation of the quoted person, obtain these in good time so that they do not delay submission.

■ Personal websites

If you have a personal website and want to post your work there, you need to check the copyright or licensing conditions first. If you published under a **Creative Commons licence**, there are no restrictions on what you may post on your own, non-commercial website but you need to check the precise type of CC licence if this might be considered commercial use (e.g. promoting your business). If you transferred copyright to the publisher you need to check the journal's permissions policy. Some journals allow authors to post PDFs on personal websites, others allow only a pre-final non-formatted version to be posted (e.g. a Word document of the copy edited accepted, revised manuscript), while others restrict authors to posting a link to the publisher's website. A handy site for checking publishers' self-archiving policies is **SHERPA/RoMEO**.

See also **web publication/institutional websites**.

■ Pharmaceutical Research and Manufacturers of America (PhRMA)

If you are working for or with a US drug company you should be aware of the PhRMA *Principles on Conduct of Clinical Trials and Communication of Clinical Trial Results* which were issued in 2002 and revised in 2004, 2009 and 2014.

www.phrma.org/principles-and-guidelines-clinical-trials

■ Physician Payments Sunshine Act; *see* Sunshine Act

■ Pico / PICO

This term has two meanings relevant to publications:

1. *The BMJ* uses it in the sense of indicating something very small (as in picomolar) to describe the short, one-page articles (akin to extended abstracts, and running to about 550 words) that it publishes in the print and iPad versions of

the journal. You do not need to prepare a pico version for your initial submission to *The BMJ*, but if your article is accepted, you will need to write one, using a template supplied by the journal.

www.bmj.com/about-bmj/resources-authors/bmj-pico

2. the acronym PICO stands for Population (or Patients), Intervention, Control and Outcome and is a handy mnemonic for the elements to include in the title of articles describing controlled clinical trials. It may also be used when formulating a question or hypothesis for a study.

■ Placeholder abstracts

Some meetings accept abstracts that describe the design of a study but not the results. This can be tempting if the submission deadline is long before the meeting and you are confident of having exciting findings to present. However, there are several dangers in submitting a placeholder. The first is that many meetings will simply reject such abstracts, so you will have wasted your time. The second is that, despite careful planning, you may not actually have results in time for the meeting. The third is that your results spring surprises so that **key players** cannot agree on their meaning in time for the meeting. Less scrupulous companies have sometimes withdrawn abstracts if results proved unfavourable, but this practice is unacceptable, since it constitutes **selective publication** and contributes to **publication bias**.

A better strategy is to submit to meetings with more convenient deadlines, or those that accept **late breaker abstracts**.

■ Plagiarism

In science one may progress, like Sir Isaac Newton, by 'standing on the shoulders of giants' but you should not conceal the acrobatics. In other words, it is acceptable (in fact, essential) to reference other works, but you must always acknowledge them and you should never copy sections from other publications and pass them off as your own work.

The Committee on Publication Ethics states 'all sources should be disclosed, and if large amounts of other people's written or illustrative material is to be used, permission must be sought'. *See* **permissions** for more details.

Remember that, in many cases, the author does not hold the **copyright** to work published in a journal or book. In such cases, strictly speaking, you will need permission to reproduce substantial sections of your own work. In practice, this certainly means obtaining permission to reproduce figures or tables.

Leaving aside the ethical and legal arguments, plagiarism (even self-plagiarism) is a sign of lazy writing. Every publication should have a unique **key message** and bolting together bits of other papers is not the most effective way of getting this across. If you need to describe a standard method it is usually better (and shorter) to reference the original work. If you are tempted to copy parts of other papers because you are not writing in your native language, you will produce a better paper if you write down your own ideas, however ungrammatical, and then ask a native speaker to edit them.

If you believe somebody has plagiarised your work you should alert your publisher before considering contacting the author or the publisher of the stolen version. One advantage of publishers holding the copyright of your work is that they are usually prepared to defend your case and advise you how to proceed.

Further reading:

Wager E (2014) Defining and responding to plagiarism. *Learn Publ.* **27**: 33–42.

■ Planning

See Chapter 2 'Developing a publication plan for a multicentre study' (pp. 7–11) and Chapter 3 'How long will it take?' (pp. 13–17) for more details of this essential aspect of getting research published.

Remember that you need an agreed strategy before you can start to plan. Also, that the more detailed the plan (in terms of publication milestones and who is responsible for doing what), the more likely it is to be realistic and helpful. If you are working to tight deadlines (e.g. to get an abstract submitted) you should circulate the plan to all key players to make sure they can meet the timelines (e.g. they are not planning a holiday around crucial dates). If timelines change, keep everybody informed. If you are trying to coordinate multiple publications (e.g. developing a product publication strategy), you might consider appointing a project manager whose sole responsibility is keeping the projects on track. In other cases, the lead author or professional writer can perform this role; but remember that being a brilliant scientist or communicator does not automatically make somebody a wonderful project manager.

■ Platinum Open Access

A term used to describe the happy (but, sadly, quite rare) situation in which journals are fully Open Access but don't levy **article processing charges**. This ideal world for authors (and funders) is usually made possible by an organisation sponsoring a journal. Also called **Diamond Open Access**.

■ Pooled data

A form of **secondary publication** using data from more than one study. Only data from published studies should be included, since it is important that the methods of each included study have been reported in full, so that readers can judge whether the pooling is appropriate and valid. If several studies are run in different regions (e.g. Europe, Asia, North America) with identical or similar protocols it may make sense to pool the results, but, as with any secondary analysis, caution and statistical advice are recommended.

■ PLOS; *see* Public Library of Science

■ Poster presentations

Abstracts submitted to conferences may be accepted for either oral or poster presentations. If the conference allows you to state a preference for oral or poster presentation this should form part of your publication strategy. Posters are generally considered less prestigious than oral presentations but may be better if you lack confidence in spoken English. Another advantage of presenting work as a poster is that you can distribute copies of the poster at the meeting and send them to people who need to know the results. (Copies of posters are usually more informative than copies of slide sets.) However, you should avoid distributing copies of posters to journalists or widely to people who did not attend the conference or were not involved in the study, since extensive reporting of research could jeopardise full publication in a journal.

Preparing a successful poster is an art. Many companies and large institutions have design departments who can do this, or, if you have a budget, you can hire a graphic designer. While professionally prepared posters look attractive, they should not resemble promotional material. A discreet logo is acceptable, and maybe even using colours associated with a product, institution or company, but posters should be regarded as scientific communications and therefore should not make excessive use of brand names or other promotional devices. Reserve your creative talents for deciding how to present your data so that your **key messages** are rapidly and clearly communicated. Remember that most conference participants spend only a couple of minutes scanning each poster. Logical organisation, clear graphics and good use of colour can help get your message across.

Like slide sets and anything submitted to journals, ensure plenty of time for everybody to comment on the poster layout and content, and then allow sufficient time for poster production. Getting agreement on the draft contents before a professional designer starts work will help to keep your design costs within budget and avoid expensive and time-consuming amendments.

Conferences usually provide information about the size and orientation of posters. If you are working to a strict budget, get agreement on the number of handouts, whether these are colour or black and white, and check on different production methods (e.g. one large sheet or separate sections, laminated or not) that will affect production costs. If you have to take a poster to a distant meeting think about airline baggage restrictions. If you do not want to risk consigning the poster to the hold (where it could get lost or damaged) you will need a format that can be carried as hand baggage. Some companies can print a poster on fabric so you can fold it and put it in your pocket.

Posters displayed for a few days at meetings are generally not considered permanent publications. However, conference organisers may make posters available on their website and *F1000Research* will publish posters. Aware that poster publication might be considered **'prior publication'**, and thus frowned upon by some journals, F1000 polled major publishers and received an interesting range of opinions on this. For example, Elsevier said that publishing a poster wouldn't prevent you from publishing a full paper in one of its journals, Lippincott Williams and Wilkins said it definitely would prevent publication, and Springer said it depended on the journal. Since *F1000Research* does not peer review posters, they may be considered like **preprints**, and you can check journals' preprint policies on **SHERPA/RoMEO** (www.sherpa.ac.uk/romeo/).

Fraser J, Fuller L, Hutber G (2009) *Creating Effective Conference Abstracts and Posters in Biomedicine.* Radcliffe Publishing, Oxford.

■ Post-publication comments

Back in the good old days of ink on dead trees, the most comments authors could expect was perhaps one or two **letters to the editor** published, in a leisurely sort of way, several months after their article, to which they might be invited to respond. Now, in the hectic world of electronic publishing, some journals encourage readers to comment, annotate and even rate articles and *PLOS One* goes so far as to describe itself as an interactive journal. If your work has been published in a journal with a rapid-response facility, it is a good idea to set up an alert to tell you when comments have been posted. It is also a good idea to agree with your co-authors about how you will respond to such comments.

■ Post-publication peer review

Traditionally, peer review occurs before publication; however, some journals, notably *F1000Research*, offer post-publication peer review (i.e. articles are published as soon as they are submitted and then peer reviewed and revised). *F1000Research* invites reviewers in the normal way but other journals have experimented with public review, in which articles are posted on a journal website as soon as they are submitted and anybody may comment on them. The idea (which sounds great in theory) is that public-spirited and highly qualified readers would point out flaws in papers and authors could respond by revising their papers. This would save editors the hard work of finding reviewers and also sounds wonderfully transparent and democratic. A couple of journals have experimented with this system but found it unworkable, as few readers posted any comments and those that did weren't particularly helpful. Another problem with the system is that authors were reluctant to allow their articles to appear on a public website before they were accepted by a journal because they feared that this would prevent them from being considered by many other journals. *See also* **prior publication**.

Wager E (2009) If comment is cheap, why is peer review so expensive? *The BMJ* blog. http://blogs.bmj.com/bmj/2009/04/16/

Smith R (2011) A woeful tale of the uselessness of peer review. *The BMJ* blog. http://blogs. bmj.com/bmj/2011/11/11/richard-smith-a-woeful-tale-of-the-uselessness-of-peer-review/

Peer review trial and debate (2006). *Nature.* **442**: xiii.

■ Predatory journals; *see* predatory publishers

■ Predatory publishers

These are companies that set up electronic journals which claim to be peer reviewed and even, in some cases, indexed, but, in fact, will publish virtually anything so long as the authors pay an **article processing charge**. They recruit authors by sending 'spam' e-mails to thousands of researchers inviting them to submit to their journals or to edit a special issue. Many of these companies hide their true location (e.g. claiming to be based in the USA when actually working from Asia), are not transparent about the fees they charge, and misrepresent their review processes. One way to check whether a journal or publisher is a predator is to consult **Beall's list**. Another way is simply to check what the journal has published and to check whether they really are included in the indexes they claim (by trying to find them in the indexes). Some of these journals aim to attract academics who need to produce publications in journals with an impact factor by quoting bogus **impact factors**.

The activities of predatory publishers were nicely shown by investigative journalist John Bohannon, who submitted over 300 fake, and clearly flawed, articles to Open Access journals, over half of which accepted them for publication.[1]

Be wary of any journal (or conference) you have never heard of that solicits contributions via e-mail. Always make a thorough check of their website and previous publications. If in doubt, consult Beall's list. Of course, many **Open Access** journals are highly reputable (Bohannon noted that *PLOS One* rejected his spoof manuscript promptly, without peer review, on ethical grounds) but predatory publishers have increased alarmingly in recent years so authors need to be cautious. The danger of falling prey to a predatory publisher is that the journal is likely to disappear without trace, probably won't be indexed, and therefore your research will not be visible to potential readers.

1 Bohannon J (2013) Who's afraid of peer review? *Science.* **342**: 60–5.

■ Preprints

Preprints are early versions of manuscripts that are posted on a public website before or without peer review. In some disciplines, notably physics, posting early versions of research papers on repositories and specialised preprint servers such as Arxiv (http://arxiv.org/) is the norm and doesn't necessarily prevent subsequent publication in a peer-reviewed journal. However, most medical journals will not consider articles that have already been posted on public websites. As ever, you need to check your target journal before you post anything as policies do vary (e.g. *The BMJ* and *PLOS Medicine* will consider articles that have appeared as preprints, but *JAMA* and *The Lancet* will not). The easiest way to find journals' preprint policies is on **SHERPA/RoMEO**. A few journals in biology and medicine, e.g. *PeerJ*, offer preprint functions themselves (i.e. authors can opt to make their article available before or without peer review). This may sound attractive if you want your article to be available quickly, but you need to consider the consequences if it is not accepted. *F1000Research* posts articles on its website before they are peer reviewed and revised, thus creating a type of temporary preprint; however, *F1000Research* claims it is not a preprint server because the articles have **DOI**s, are considered fully published, and may not be submitted to another journal if they are not accepted.

■ Press conferences

If you (or your company or institution) want to hold a press conference to announce a publication you must let the journal know. Most editors are delighted by opportunities to publicise work appearing in their journals but you should always liaise closely with the journal or publisher's press department.

Major meetings sometimes invite authors to attend press conferences to talk about their presentations. This can cause problems if your work has already been accepted by a journal with a strict **embargo** policy, so always check with the journal before agreeing.

See also the sections on **media relations** and **press releases**.

■ Press releases

A press release about research is fine if you issue it in consultation with a journal or meeting but potentially hazardous to the health of your publication if you issue it independently. Journal editors do not like authors talking to the press before an article is published and they particularly dislike results being discussed in newspapers, or on the radio or television, before they appear in the peer-reviewed literature. However, these same editors are delighted by media attention when papers are published. The rule for authors is simple: once your paper has been accepted for publication, do not contact the press without agreement from the journal.

Press interest in meeting presentations can cause problems since this takes place before the full version is published and could, in theory, jeopardise full publication if mishandled. However, most journals appreciate that journalists attend major meetings and accept that preliminary findings may therefore get reported. The general rule is that, if you are questioned by the press you should provide no more detail than appears in the abstract, since this is already in the public domain. You should not provide copies of slides, the wording of your talk or extended abstracts. To be on the safe side, you probably should not provide copies of posters to journalists, since these can contain considerable detail. This might seem odd, since attendees at the meeting can see (and photograph) your poster, and you can hand out copies (and even post it on a conference website or *F1000Research*), so you might consider the poster to be as much in the public domain as the abstract. However, to avoid detailed reports appearing in the press and jeopardising your chance of full publication in a peer-reviewed journal, this is the safest strategy.

Perhaps surprisingly, most journals do not consider a 'webcast' (i.e. posting a video of a presentation) from a meeting to constitute prior publication.[1]

1 For example: Kassirer JP (1999) Posting presentations at medical meetings on the internet. *N Engl J Med*. **340**: 803.

■ Pre-submission enquiries

Some editors welcome pre-submission enquiries from authors seeking guidance about whether their journal is the right place for a particular piece of work or type of publication. If a journal website offers this facility give it a try, but if it does not you may simply be told to submit your article in the usual way and wait for a response. Pre-submission enquiries are especially helpful if you want to submit something that the journal generally commissions (such as an editorial, commentary or book review) or if you are planning something that does not fit into the normal publication categories or is not the type of thing that the journal normally publishes (e.g. a meeting report or set of guidelines). Some journals require pre-submission enquiries only for this sort of article (e.g. *JAMA* requires them for reviews and special communications).

A few journals (notably *PLOS Medicine*)[1] always require authors to submit a covering letter and abstract before going on to a full submission. However, other journals work differently. *The BMJ* notes 'it is not always possible for us to answer all presubmission inquiries' so they have produced a checklist[2] to help authors decide whether *The BMJ* is the right place for their work (which a well-placed informant tells me is known as the 'reject-your-own-paper' page).

1 http://journals.plos.org/plosmedicine/s/presubmission-inquiries

2 www.bmj.com/about-bmj/resources-authors/forms-policies-and-checklists/bmj-right-journal-my-research-article

■ Primary publication

If a single study produces several publications they are usually classified into primary and secondary. The primary publication is the one that presents the main findings of the study in full for the first time. Primary publications usually follow the **Introduction, Methods, Results and Discussion (IMRAD)** structure and report the study's primary outcome(s). There might be more than one primary publication (e.g. presenting clinical and economic aspects of a trial) but this is unusual. Since the primary publication should include a detailed description of the research methods, and since readers will need to understand the methods in order to evaluate the findings, having a single paper, or linked papers in the same journal issue, will avoid duplication. If you are developing more than one paper from a single piece of research you should indicate this when you submit any of the papers for publication. It is good practice to include copies of related papers (or manuscripts) in your submission package to reassure the editor that there is not too much overlap or redundancy. Linked papers should be clearly cross-referenced.

Secondary publications (e.g. sub-group analyses and follow-up studies) should not appear before the primary publication and should always reference it. Your publication strategy should take this into account, especially if you plan to publish your primary paper in a prestigious journal with long acceptance and/or **lead times** and a secondary paper in a journal that happens to be more rapid.

It is important to distinguish primary from secondary publications to avoid 'double-counting' in reviews and meta-analyses. For example, if data from an interim analysis, 6-month follow-up and 5-year follow-up are published without clear study identification or cross-referencing, the same patients could be included up to three times in a meta-analysis. Since the population characteristics (number of patients, mean age, etc.) will, by definition, differ for each analysis, it can be surprisingly difficult to determine whether the papers report the same study. Including a trial registration number should help reduce confusion when several papers report findings from the same study. To avoid 'double-counting' it is also important to cross-reference **translations** of primary papers clearly to the original publication.

■ Prior publication

Most peer-reviewed journals will consider only work that has not previously been published in full (this is sometimes referred to as the **'Ingelfinger rule'**). Some journals require authors to state this in their covering letter or to sign a declaration that this is the case. If you want to get your work published, you therefore need to avoid the pitfall of 'prior publication'. The **International Committee of Medical Journal Editors' (ICMJE)** guidelines available at www.icmje.org provide some useful definitions.

In simple terms, **abstracts**, **posters** and **oral presentations** do not constitute prior publication. However, extended abstracts (>500 words) or conference proceedings sometimes do.

Presenting results at internal (company or institution) meetings, or to trial investigators, participants or regulators should not affect later publication. However, circulating a research report to a wide audience not involved with the study might cause problems.

Posting preliminary (unreviewed) reports on websites is currently a grey area. Some journals consider that this is analogous to presenting findings at a meeting, and are not bothered by the appearance of so-called **preprints**.[1] Others take a much firmer line and consider them to be prior publications. Disciplines outside medicine (notably physics) have used preprint servers such as Arxiv for some time and these seem to exist happily alongside the peer-reviewed journals.

Since September 2008, under the **FDAAA** legislation, US law has required that result summaries of trials of new drugs that will be sold in the USA must be posted on **ClinicalTrials.gov**. This initially caused concern about whether such postings would constitute **prior publication** (and therefore prevent later publication in a peer-reviewed journal). However, the **ICMJE** announced that posting the summary tables required by FDAAA would not affect publication in a journal, but, they have warned that more extensive release of results via other websites might.

Some journals ask authors to list previous presentations at meetings. This might help readers trying to link abstracts with full papers, which can sometimes be surprisingly tricky. For more on this subject, *see* **trial identifier**.

1   For example: Delamothe T, Smith R, Keller MA *et al.* (1999) Netprints: the next phase in the evolution of biomedical publishing. *BMJ.* **319**: 1515–16.

Marusić A and Huić M (2008) Registration of clinical trials still moving ahead – September 2008 update to uniform requirements for manuscripts submitted to biomedical journals. *Croat Med J.* **49**: 582–5.

■ PRISMA

Guidelines on the Preferred Reporting Items for Systematic Reviews and Meta-Analyses (PRISMA). These guidelines replaced QUOROM (which stood for Quality Of Reporting Of Meta-analyses but often got misspelled as 'quorum'). They are similar to **CONSORT** (for randomised trials) and **STROBE** (for epidemiological research), and, like them, are available on the **EQUATOR Network** website. Useful if you are writing up a systematic review.

www.prisma-statement.org/

■ Promoting your work

Journals are happy for authors (and sponsors) to promote their work. In the old days, the only channels available were **press releases**, printed **reprints**, citations in later work and word of mouth. Now, journals may encourage authors to provide multimedia offerings such as video clips, podcasts and slide sets. Journals as well as authors are also increasingly likely to use **social media** such as **blogs** and Twitter to announce and discuss publications and encourage people to read them.

Pharmaceutical companies must comply with national and regional regulations since many activities that go beyond publishing in traditional peer-reviewed journals and presenting at scientific meetings may be viewed as marketing. However, since many of these new media options have emerged only recently, legislation and guidelines may lag behind the technology, so careful interpretation may be required to predict how the regulators may react.

Some publishers are experimenting with methods for highlighting, bundling and rating published work. Journals may tag highly downloaded articles, create topic streams or theme issues, or allow readers to rate articles. If you value these features and believe they will benefit your article, you should seek out journals that offer them or if, like the rest of us, you remain confused or cynical, you can ignore them or regard them as an unexpected bonus (or setback).

■ Proofs (page proofs)

Journals send proofs (usually via e-mail) to the corresponding author shortly before publication and often expect these to be checked and returned in a short space of time. For most articles you will receive page proofs, i.e. laid out as the pages will appear in the journal, with figures correctly placed, headers and footers according to journal style, etc. **Galley proofs** (i.e. single columns of text not made up into pages) are almost obsolete except for letters or 'filler' items which get squeezed into issues just before publication.

To prevent delays it is important that the **corresponding author** can be reached and can respond quickly. Although some people believe that being the corresponding author indicates some level of merit or seniority (perhaps equating it with the **guarantor**), in practical terms it makes sense to select someone who will be available and likely to handle reviewer comments and proofs efficiently.

Use of conventional proofreading symbols will increase the chances that corrections will be made as you intended. You can find proofreading marks at: www. journalismcareers.com/articles/proofreadingsymbols.shtml.

When reading proofs remember that your article will probably have been put into the journal's **house style**. There is no point in resisting such changes and requesting that everything be put back to how you originally wrote it. However, if a copy editor has changed your meaning or introduced errors, you may correct this. If you discover major problems with the proofs it is best to contact the journal to discuss them.

The corresponding author should agree with the other authors, in advance, how the proofs will be handled. There may not be time (or it may not achieve much) to circulate proofs to all authors but, if possible, proofs should be checked by at least two people. Proofreading is when **nitpickers** can be really useful as they often spot mistakes that others miss and may actually enjoy the process.

■ Protocol review

Some journals review and publish research protocols before studies are completed. However, this practice has not been widely adopted so if you want your protocol reviewed this may limit your choice of **target journals**. Protocol review has several advantages for researchers. Journals that review protocols sometimes guarantee to publish the findings if the study is completed satisfactorily or at least guarantee that it will undergo external review rather than being rejected after only in-house review. Alternatively, if your protocol is rejected you know there is no point in submitting the results to that journal. If a reviewer spots a flaw in your study design it may not be too late to rectify it. Lastly, publication of the protocol might alert potential participants to the study, which could assist recruitment. Some **Open Access** journals offer a discount on the **article processing charge** if the protocol and article are published in the same journal.

From the journal's (and readers') viewpoint, protocol review offers perhaps the most impartial method of scrutinising a study's design, since the reviewer cannot be influenced by the findings. Publishing the protocol may also prevent **data dredging** or authors presenting post hoc analyses as if they were planned.

Some journals (e.g. *The BMJ*, *The Lancet*, *JAMA* and *PLOS Medicine*) require a copy of the protocol to be submitted with any paper reporting a clinical trial.

Godlee F (2001) Publishing study protocols: making them visible will improve registration, reporting and recruitment. *BMC News and Views* **2**: 4. www.biomedcentral.com/content/pdf/1471-8219-2-4.pdf

■ Publication agreements

Agreeing plans for a publication in writing, as early as possible, can avoid much misunderstanding and wrangling later. **GPP3** recommends that publication agreements for company-sponsored studies should confirm that investigators will have access to the data and will be free to publish the results and that the authors will be responsible for all final decisions on publication content. The guidelines also recommend that sponsor companies should provide authors with a copy of their **publication policy**.

Battisti W, Wager E, Baltzer L *et al.* (2015) Good Publication Practice for communicating company-sponsored medical research: GPP3. *Ann Intern Med* **163**: doi: 10.7326/M15-0288.

■ Publication bias

Publication bias occurs when studies with unfavourable findings (either in terms of the sponsor's product or the investigator's pet theory) or those with equivocal results are less likely to be published than those with favourable or positive results. Such bias is further emphasised when positive studies get published more than once, creating **redundant publications**. Some cases of non-publication and covert redundant publication have been well publicised and have resulted in bad publicity for the perpetrators.

Publication bias can skew the results of systematic reviews and meta-analyses. For this reason, such reviews sometimes include an estimate of publication bias, e.g. a funnel plot.

Various strategies to prevent or reduce publication bias have been discussed by journal editors. One is the requirement to register all trials at their inception. The members of the **International Committee of Medical Journal Editors (ICMJE)** have made **trial registration** a requirement for publication in their journals since 2005. The latest versions of the Declaration of Helsinki also call on doctors to publish the results of all research, regardless of whether they are positive or negative; this principle is also emphasized in **GPP3**.

A well-planned publication strategy should prevent publication bias by ensuring that all studies get published and that redundant publications are not created.

Chalmers I (1990) Underreporting research is scientific misconduct. *JAMA*. **263**: 1405–8.

Melander H, Ahlqvist-Rastad J, Meijer G *et al.* (2003) Evidence b(i)ased medicine – selective reporting from studies sponsored by pharmaceutical industry: review of studies in new drug applications. *BMJ*. **326**: 1171–3.

Tramèr MR, Reynolds DJM, Moore RA *et al.* (1997) Impact of covert duplicate publication on meta-analysis: a case study. *BMJ*. **315**: 635–40.

■ Publication Plan, The

A really useful free website providing information and news for people involved with publication planning and the development of medical publications. Definitely worth a look.

www.thepublicationplan.com

■ Publication policy

Any organisation that gets involved with publications ought to have a publication policy. This should set out general principles and reflect relevant guidelines (such as those from the **ICMJE** and **GPP**). Policies, unlike detailed publication strategies, can be public documents, should be applied in all cases and should only need updating when external guidelines change or new issues arise. In contrast, publication strategies and plans are usually internal documents relating to one product or project and require constant updating to reflect the progress of publications.

Helpful policies will include enough detail to inform decisions and avoid platitudes and meaningless management-speak such as 'Heavenly Pharmaceuticals will pro-actively engage in responsible publication practices that will advance the cause of science' (which doesn't really tell you anything).

Publication policies should cover topics such as authorship criteria, data ownership and access, managing and disclosing conflicts of interest as well as general statements about what will be published (e.g. a commitment to publish results of all clinical trials in peer-reviewed journals).

Drug company policies may need to reflect any **corporate integrity agreements** imposed on the company by the US regulators. Funders' policies may include requirements to publish in certain types of journal (e.g. **Open Access**).

■ Publication steering committee

This is usually just a posh term for a **writing group**. However, for big projects that will generate many publications, it can be helpful to have an overall steering committee to oversee the planning and strategy while each publication will have its own writing group.

Some drug companies appoint a publication steering committee for each product or major trial. This group takes strategic decisions such as how many publications to develop, where to present and publish them and who the authors should be. The committee is mainly or exclusively comprised of non-company personnel. Each publication then has its own writing group, which includes all the named authors and often several company employees (e.g. statisticians and medical writers).

GPP3 notes that publication steering committees should be formed early in the life of a study, before results are available, and that all investigators should be informed about the committee's membership and responsibilities. The guidelines also note that membership of a publication steering committee does not automatically qualify somebody as an author – for that, they need to fulfil recognised **authorship** criteria (e.g. those of the ICMJE).

■ Publication strategy

If you produce a publication strategy document it should fit neatly between your organisation's publication policy and detailed plans for individual publications. However, if you are only dealing with a few publications you might prefer to combine the latter two into a strategic plan – but don't forget that even the simplest publication will work better if you do have a **strategy** (i.e. an idea of where you want to end up). It can also be easier to get agreement among authors if you start by discussing the strategy in general terms and then consider the details in the plan. Since strategies and plans can merge, there is sometimes confusion about the differences so the following table sets out some general rules.

	Publication policy	*Publication strategy*	*Publication plan*
Applies to	All situations (no exceptions)	A group of publications (and may be revised)	One or more publications (and is frequently revised)
Document is usually	External	Internal – but shared with key people	Internal
Needs updating	Every few years/if external guidelines change	If strategy changes or new data become available	Frequently (to reflect progress of publications)
Refers to/ consistent with	External guidelines (e.g. ICMJE)	Internal strategies (e.g. marketing plans)	Publication strategy

For example, the publication policy might state that the company will endeavour to publish results of all clinical trials in peer-reviewed journals. The strategy for a particular study might be to publish one primary paper in a general medical journal and a sub-group analysis in a specialist European gastroenterology journal. The plan would set out the key messages for each paper, the proposed authors, the target audience, the target journal, back-up journals and target dates for publication milestones.

See **strategy** and Chapters 1–3 for more details.

■ Public Library of Science (PLOS)

PLOS describes itself as 'a nonprofit publisher and advocacy organization founded to accelerate progress in science and medicine by leading a transformation in research communication'. It publishes several **Open Access** journals including the highly selective *PLOS Medicine* and the **'mega-journal'** *PLOS One*, which was one of the first journals to use peer review only to correct errors and check that the research and reporting were sound rather than to select articles according to their potential interest level. Publishing over 30 000 papers per year, *PLOS One* is the world's largest journal. See www.plos.org.

■ PubMed

A website run by the US National Library of Medicine which gives access to **Medline** and **PubMed Central**. A useful (and free) resource for searching the literature, checking **MeSH** headings for **key words** and finding out whether a journal is included in **Medline**. The address is: www.ncbi.nlm.nih.gov/PubMed.

■ PubMed Central

An electronic archive of full-text journal articles launched by the US National Library of Medicine in 2000. Articles include those from fully **Open Access** journals and others from conventional publishers that release research papers after a set period (usually 6 to 24 months after publication). It can be searched via the PubMed website (which also gives access to **Medline**): www.ncbi.nlm.nih.gov/pmc/index.html.

Not to be confused with **BioMed Central** which is a commercial company (now part of Springer Nature) that publishes a range of Open Access journals, all of which are available on PubMed Central.

■ PubStrat

Commercial publication planning tools including a journal selector. See http://pubstrat.com/.

Q

■ Queries

It may seem obvious, but getting a prompt and helpful answer to a query depends on addressing it to the right person or department. Unfortunately, journal functions are often divided between different organisations and companies, so this is not always as straightforward as it might seem. Check the title page or website for contact telephone numbers and e-mail addresses, and to try to unravel who does what. Large, independent journals (like the '**Big Five**') tend to organise everything under one roof, whereas journals edited by academics and produced by publishers on behalf of academic societies often work out of several locations and can therefore be harder to pin down.

Use the following table as a guide to where you should direct your queries.

Query about	Large, independent journals	Smaller, 'academic' journals
Receipt of manuscript	Editorial Department	The Editor/where you submitted the manuscript
When to expect decision	Editorial Department	The Editor/where you submitted the manuscript
Appealing a decision	The Editor	The Editor

(continued)

Query about	Large, independent journals	Smaller, 'academic' journals
Serious complaint	The Editor, then **Ombudsman** (if there is one) or Editor's employer	The Editor, then the parent organisation/academic society
When to expect proofs	Journal's Production Department/Assistant Editor assigned to manuscript	Production Department (Publisher)
Query on proofs	Journal's Production Department/Assistant Editor assigned to manuscript/Technical Editor	Production Department (Publisher)
Ordering offprints/reprints	Reprint Department	Publisher/Reprint Department
Permission to reproduce figure,* etc.	Journal's Permissions Department/Publisher	Permissions Department (Publisher)
Readership	Journal's Advertising Department	Advertising Department (Publisher)

*Note: If the original was published in an Open Access journal under a Creative Commons licence you do not need permission to reuse it, but always check the journal's website.

■ Queues

Printed journals that operate within a strict **page budget** and get their money from annual subscriptions can publish only a certain number of papers in each issue. If the editor accepts more papers than the journal can publish, a queue will form. This explains the lengthy **lead time** between acceptance and publication for some journals (over a year in some cases). If speed of publication is important to you, try to discover the lead time of your **target journal**. If you simply want to cite your publication, speed of decision may be more important (since you can cite an article as 'in press' once it is accepted). If you need **offprints** by a certain date (e.g. for a particular event), contact the journal for details of their production schedule and to see if you can negotiate something to meet your needs.

Many journals make accepted material available online before it appears in print, and it may even be indexed on Medline as an '**epub** ahead of print', but there may still be some delay between acceptance and electronic publication to allow for **technical editing**.

R

■ Readership

See also **target audience**. The best place to get detailed information about the readership of a journal that carries advertisements is the **advertising department** because they use this information to persuade companies to advertise in their journal. For other journals, check the website, which may tell you who the journal is aimed at, and also any affiliations to academic societies which may give further clues. Traditional, subscription-based journals cater for a specific readership who rely on the journal to select the most relevant and interesting articles for them. In contrast, Open Access **mega-journals** expect readers to find individual articles via indexes, key words and search engines, so their readership is less well defined. Even if you are aiming for a mega-journal, it is helpful to keep your target audience in mind when you are writing as this will help to focus the paper and decide what you need to include.

■ Redundant publication

The **International Committee of Medical Journal Editors (ICMJE)** defines redundant publication as anything that overlaps substantially with another publication. The term 'duplicate publication' is sometimes used synonymously, but this may not be strictly accurate, since perpetrators do not necessarily limit themselves to only two publications and the publications may not be exact duplicates. Strict word limits in some journals, or the desire to increase one's publication list, may tempt authors to split their findings into several papers; extreme cases are condemned as **salami slicing**. However, such multiple publication may be acceptable if different parts of the study are understandable by themselves and relevant to different audiences. Some journals offer guidance on how much overlap is acceptable, but this is a grey area. *The BMJ* notes that 'Whenever an article ... overlaps by more than 10% with previously published work, or work submitted elsewhere, we expect authors to send us copies of those articles'.

Journal editors frown on redundant publication because they prefer to publish original, rather than recycled, material. They may also be concerned that undetected duplication may skew the results of systematic reviews and meta-analyses. Extensive repetition may also breach copyright. The key to preventing such **publication bias** is clear **trial identifiers**. Secondary analyses, follow-up studies and **translations** should be clearly labelled as such and should always include a reference to the original study.

Companies that have invested heavily in a major study will, understandably, want to get the most out of publications if the findings are favourable. (Although, interestingly, a survey of duplicate publications found that only 33% were sponsored by the pharmaceutical industry, so perhaps academic pressures create an even greater temptation.[1]) However, a responsible publication strategy should not include any redundant publications. If the moral argument is not enough, remember that detection of deliberate redundant publication can bring negative publicity and duplicate articles may be retracted (*see* references for examples). Worse still, almost 70% of journal editors said they would impose restrictions on future submissions for any author found guilty of redundant publication.[2]

Guidance on the acceptability of repeated or **'encore' abstracts** is less clear-cut than that for journals and some conferences will accept them.

1 von Elm E, Poglia G, Walder B *et al.* (2004) Different patterns of duplicate publication: an analysis of articles used in systematic reviews. *JAMA.* **291**: 974–80.

2 Yank V and Barnes D (2003) Consensus and contention regarding redundant publications in clinical research: cross-sectional survey of editors and authors. *J Med Ethics.* **29**: 109–14.

Huston P and Moher D (1996) Redundancy, disaggregation, and the integrity of medical research. *Lancet.* **347**: 1024–6.

Tramèr MR, Reynolds DJM, Moore RA *et al.* (1997) Impact of covert duplicate publication on meta-analysis: a case study. *BMJ.* **315**: 635–40.

Horton R (2008) Retraction – a growing, bleeding, violet mole. *Lancet.* **371**: 288.

■ References

Preparing references can be a tedious job and numerous studies show that reference lists frequently contain errors. One common cause is copying citations from other papers without reading the actual reference. Although it still falls short of perfection, you should at least obtain an abstract and check the reference from **Medline** or the journal website, but, of course, you should really read the full article. If you don't have access to the full text and can't afford (or resent paying) to download it, you could try **DeepDyve** which allows you to rent an article for 24 hours. The best way to overcome the drudgery of typing references and reformatting them is to invest in **bibliographic software** such as Reference Manager or EndNote or free programs such as Mendeley (which can also organise your PDF files).

Even if you have prepared the reference list with great care, it is easy to omit a detail or make a typing mistake. Queries about references tend to be spotted by technical editors rather than reviewers and therefore come at the proof stage, when you are in a hurry and facing a deadline. It is a good habit to make (or scan) a copy of the first page of every reference cited in a paper and file these with the typescript. This will save a lot of frantic scrabbling about (and may therefore avoid delays) if you need to check a reference later.

■ Reformatting

If your paper is rejected by your **target journal**, you should check the instructions of your **second target journal** and reformat the typescript so that it complies. The reference section is usually the most time-consuming to reformat, unless you have used **bibliographic software** to create your reference list, in which case this task will be quick and easy. The other section that often needs adjustment is the abstract, since different journals have different requirements for structure and length.

If you do not reformat your submission you may reduce your chance of acceptance because the reviewer or editor may assume that you could not be bothered to meet the journal's requirements, or (rightly) that the paper has been rejected by another journal. The former is probably worse than the latter. Most editors of specialist journals realise that they have higher acceptance rates than prestigious general journals so a previous rejection should not count against you. Some journals even request copies of previous reviews, and if a review for a general journal praises your work but suggests it is of specialist interest, the second editor may decide it does not need further review, so this can work in the authors' favour.

Reflecting the waste of effort that repeated reformatting represents, *PeerJ* and some Elsevier journals will consider submissions in any format and only require authors to do detailed formatting for the specific journal style after acceptance. Sadly, this policy doesn't yet apply to all of Elsevier's medical journals, or to those from other publishers, but let's hope this sensible and author-friendly approach catches on.

Fennell C and Barrie R (2014) 'Your Paper, Your Way' simplifies submissions. Elsevier blog. www.elsevier.com/authors-update/story/online-submissionpeer-review/your-paper-your-way-simplifies-papers-submission

■ Rejection

■ Rates

Rejection rates range from around 20% for many non-selective (or **'mega'**) **journals** (such as *PLOS One*) to over 90% for prestigious, general journals (such as the **'Big Five'**). If speed of publication is important, you need to select your target journal carefully, since a string of rejections will delay publication as well as dent your morale. However, some journals with high rejection rates have relatively rapid **decision times** because they reject a high proportion of articles after **in-house review**. Some journals publish rejection (or acceptance) rates on their website. Rates may vary for different parts of the journal; for example short reports and research letters may have lower rejection rates than full papers. The best way to avoid rejection (as well as doing brilliant research) is to research your target journal carefully and then to follow its instructions with equal care.

■ Times

Rejection times range from a few days, for some journals that employ **in-house review** or offer **expedited review**, to several months. The worst I have experienced is 6 months. The average time if your paper undergoes external peer review is around 3 months – this is a good figure to use for planning. If you have not heard from a journal after 3 months you should politely enquire to make sure your manuscript has not been lost or forgotten. This may also spur the editor into nudging a tardy reviewer.

Times from submission to rejection tend to be shorter than those from submission to acceptance, especially for journals that reject a sizeable proportion of papers without sending them for external peer review. It may therefore be worth the risk of submitting to a journal with a high **rejection rate** if you can be fairly sure of a rapid rejection. In this case, honour will have been satisfied that you attempted to get into a high **impact factor** or prestigious journal but you will not have wasted too much time in the attempt.

However, on a gloomier note, remember that journals with high rejection rates still reject many papers after sending them out for external peer review and, in some cases (such as *The Lancet*) even after asking authors to respond to reviewers' comments. Coming close to acceptance may therefore be a worse fate than a swift, outright rejection, unless the reviewers suggest changes that will increase your chance of acceptance by another journal.

The psychological effects of rejection seem worse if you have waited a long time for a decision and it is easy to lose momentum and motivation. It is therefore vital to have a **back-up plan**.

■ Reporting guidelines

A wide range of reporting guidelines that aim to improve the reporting of medical research are available. The major guidelines have been endorsed by many journals and you may have to submit a completed checklist with your manuscript to show that it complies with the relevant guideline. Check journal instructions for specific requirements. The best place to find reporting guidelines is the EQUATOR Network website, www.equator-network.org. Even if your target journal does not require you to follow a particular guideline, it is good practice to be aware of them and try to follow them if you can, and this may increase your chance of acceptance or reduce the number of reviewers' comments you have to deal with.

■ Reprints

Strictly speaking, a reprint is a copy of an article produced after publication. The correct term for extra copies ordered at the time of publication is **offprints** (although the terms are often used interchangeably), so *see* this section for further details.

In the old days receiving reprint (or offprint) requests from far-flung spots was a pleasant by-product of publication and a good way of enhancing your stamp collection. These days, most researchers seem to have access to electronic libraries or photocopiers, so requests are rarer, but still enjoyable and are sent by e-mail, so they don't need stamps. Remember that only the corresponding author will have the pleasure of receiving requests, so it is a nice idea to keep other authors informed as everybody likes to hear that somebody actually wants to read their article.

■ Retractions

If a journal discovers that it has published a flawed or misleading paper (either because of honest error or because of scientific misconduct such as plagiarism or fraud) it may retract the paper. The notice of retraction will appear in indexing systems that cover the journal. Although, in complex studies, contributors may take responsibility for only part of the research, all authors (or contributors) will be affected by such a retraction, so think hard before putting your name on a paper if you have any doubts about it. Editors may retract articles for publication misconduct (e.g. **redundant publication**) as well as research fraud.

For more detail, see the Committee on Publication Ethics (COPE) retraction guidelines at: http://publicationethics.org/files/retraction%20guidelines.pdf.

For a lively blog on retractions and great insights into research and publication misconduct, go to http://retractionwatch.com/.

■ Reviewer choice

Some journals allow authors to suggest potential reviewers. It is hard to discover how often editors act on these suggestions, although journals that require suggestions almost certainly use them more often than those that do not. If your target journal requires reviewer suggestions, discuss potential reviewers with your co-authors and agree on your suggestions well before submission (don't leave it to the last minute). Check the journal's criteria; for example, people from the same institution and previous co-authors are usually disallowed. Remember that you usually need to supply e-mail addresses for the suggested reviewers.

Authors may also indicate if there is anybody who should be excluded from the review process (e.g. on the grounds of a strong competing interest). Again, it is difficult to know whether editors honour these requests all the time. Cynics have suggested that identifying somebody you think should not review your paper might be counterproductive, as the editor would be tempted to use this person just to ensure a really tough review. Journal editors will probably protest that they are not like that … and in fact this was the response I got to an informal survey.[1]

Some electronic submission forms have spaces for proposing or opposing reviewers. If this facility is not available and you feel strongly that an individual should not review your paper, you should mention this in your covering letter.

Editors are most likely to respect your wishes if you give a compelling (and polite) explanation, such as an insurmountable conflict of interest. Implying that the individual is mentally unstable or a cantankerous old curmudgeon will probably not advance your cause.

1 Wager E (2004) Use of author-nominated reviewers: an informal survey. *European Science Editing*. **30**: 117–18.

Wager E, Parkin EC and Tamber PS (2006) Are reviewers suggested by authors as good as those chosen by editors? Results of a rater-blinded, retrospective study. *BMC Med*. **4**: 13.

Moore A (2015) Author-suggested reviewers – Or the helper's dilemma. *BioEssays* **37**: 929.

■ Reviewers' comments

Unconditional acceptances are incredibly rare, so you will nearly always have to respond to reviewers' comments. If your work is rejected and you plan to submit it to another journal you can, of course, ignore these comments but it makes sense to swallow your pride and read them, once your disappointment has worn off, to see if they identify any obvious mistakes or ways in which you could improve your paper. (It is also possible that your second target journal will use the same reviewer as the first – in which case it is definitely preferable to have followed at least some of his or her suggestions.)

If you receive a conditional acceptance you may still need to swallow a little pride but you should consider reviewers' comments as negotiable suggestions rather than a diktat and, if you can provide good reasons, you do not have to follow them all. Hywel Williams (an experienced editor, reviewer and author) notes 'referees are not gods, but human beings who make mistakes', and goes on to suggest three golden rules: 'answer completely, answer politely and answer with evidence'.[1]

Most journals ask authors for a detailed response, either in a covering letter or a list, to show that you have responded to every point. You may also be asked to supply a copy of the paper with revisions highlighted. As well as helping the journal editor, these are useful tools for discussing revisions with co-authors. The **corresponding author** will receive the reviewers' comments, but this does not mean that s/he has to draft the entire response. It is often best to divide the questions among authors depending on their expertise. However you organise the response, make sure to involve all your **key players**, since everybody must approve the final version.

Your response should be polite and professional. Where possible, and especially if you are explaining why you have *not* made a suggested change, support your argument with evidence (e.g. references) just as you would in a paper. If reviewers request conflicting actions (e.g. to expand and cut the same section) check the editor's covering letter, which should indicate how to handle this, or contact the editor for advice. Do not forget to respond to points in the editor's letter as well as to those in the reviewers' reports. In fact, editors' requests should take priority over reviewer suggestions.

Some journals set a deadline for responding (often 4 to 6 weeks). If this causes insurmountable problems (e.g. if you have to perform extra analyses and simply cannot get them done in time) contact the editor as soon as possible to explain the situation and see if you can negotiate an extension. However, if possible, try to respond reasonably promptly. Most people find revisions vaguely dispiriting, so it is tempting to postpone this task and its prospect only gets worse the longer you procrastinate. Think positive, congratulate yourself on getting a conditional acceptance (if, indeed, you have) and consider this the penultimate stage towards your publication goal. Or bribe yourself with promises of a stiff drink/chocolate/ your favourite legal indulgence once you have resubmitted.

If you plan not to resubmit but prefer to try your luck at another journal, it is helpful to let the first journal know.

On a gloomier note, read the letter from the editor carefully. Some journals only agree to 'reconsider' your paper after you have responded to the reviewers' comments, and may reject a fair proportion after this stage. (For example, *The Lancet*'s instructions state: 'Submissions that survive in-house and peer review might be referred back to authors for revision. This is an invitation to present the best possible paper for further scrutiny by the journal; it is not an acceptance'.) Receiving a rejection after you have made revisions may seem unfair and annoying, but it is even more irksome if you have gone around telling everybody that your paper has been accepted.

Some journals ask authors to send reviewers' comments they have received from other journals. I used to think this was a rather ridiculous request, as most authors are reluctant to admit that their work has already been rejected by another journal. However, I am softening my views on this strategy, and even recommending it in some cases, since hearing that some journals will accept a publication on the basis of another journal's review, especially if the reviewers liked the paper but the editor thought it was better suited for a different type of journal. The most obvious example would be if your paper was good enough to be sent out for external review by a really top-notch general journal (like *The Lancet* or *NEJM*) and you are now submitting it to a specialist journal. Supplying reviewers' comments should also prevent a journal from sending your paper to the same reviewer again (but only if the review is signed). If you do pass reviewers' comments from one journal to another, you may also include a rebuttal explaining why you have not made all the suggested changes – but the second editor will probably expect you to have addressed at least some of the issues raised by the reviewers.

Some publishers will pass reviewer comments to a second journal (usually within the same publishing group) if the authors have signed up for this – *see* **journal cascades**.

1 Williams HC (2004) How to reply to referees' comments when submitting manuscripts for publication. *J Am Acad Dermatol.* **51**: 79–83.

Wager E. How to respond to peer reviewer comments – 10 tips for success. www.drugs incontext.com/category/resources/

■ Review process

The BMJ once included a delightful typo that changed external review into eternal review.[1] This provides a useful mnemonic for the two basic review processes and the effects they have on review speed.

Journals that have high **rejection rates** and employ a substantial editorial staff often reject up to 50% of submissions after **internal review** alone. Only those papers that the editors consider they are likely to publish are sent for review by external experts. This system means that **rejection times** tend to be much shorter than acceptance times (*see* **acceptance times** for details). It may therefore make sense to submit to such a journal even if you harbour only a slim hope of acceptance since rejection is likely to be swift.

Less well-staffed journals (i.e. those edited by academics rather than full-time editors) tend to send all submissions for **external review** and, subsequently, rejection and acceptance take about the same length of time. Journals may either use **editorial board** members or a larger database of reviewers to review papers, but this difference probably has little effect on the time to get a decision. Journals that offer rapid review may pay their reviewers.

Once the editor has received the reviewers' reports, the submission may be discussed at an editorial board or selection committee meeting, e.g. *The BMJ*'s **Hanging Committee**. If meetings are infrequent, this may increase the time to get a decision. Further delay may be caused by additional reviews, e.g. by a statistician.

Some journals ask authors to suggest potential reviewers, but (according to an informal survey that I carried out) this does not seem to increase the number of reviews obtained for each paper so it is unlikely to affect the speed of review.

1 Latham JN (2004) Just how rapid is 'eternal' review? *BMJ*. **329**: 801.

■ Role of sponsor / funding source; *see* sponsor, role of

■ RoMEO; *see* SHERPA/RoMEO

■ Running title

This is a short version of a paper's title that often appears as a header on the journal page and is usually written on the title page of a typescript. Check your target journal's instructions to see if a running title is required and, if so, how long it can be. This is one of those minor points which, if you forget it, or fail to follow the instructions, should not really affect your paper's chance of acceptance but which, especially if combined with other minor offences, is likely to annoy editors, perhaps suggest that your paper has been rejected by another journal, and generally give a poor impression. Try to include the running title on an early draft of the paper, since all authors should approve it and it may be overlooked on the pre-submission check. Condensing a title often has the effect of making it more direct, especially if it describes the study findings rather than just the study design. It is therefore important to ensure that it is justified and not over-promotional.

S

■ Salami science / slicing

This descriptive phrase, originally coined by Ed Huth, refers to the much frowned-upon practice of splitting or reanalysing data from a single study to generate as many publications as possible.[1] It probably occurs equally in academia (where researchers are judged by the length rather than the quality of their CV) and industry (where companies are keen to get positive findings published as often as possible). As with many questions in scientific publication, good judgement is required when deciding how many publications your findings warrant. In answering this question, try to keep the reader in mind and consider which results should be presented together.

As a general rule, most clinical trials generate a single, primary paper, which describes the primary outcome set out in the protocol and often some of the secondary outcomes or incidental findings. This may, legitimately, be followed by secondary papers describing sub-set analyses or follow-ups. It is common for economic findings to be presented separately from clinical ones, but *The BMJ* will not consider **economic evaluations** on their own.[2]

If you do produce more than one paper from a publication, make sure that the links are transparent (e.g. by including a **trial identifier** or registration number) and always reference the primary publication.

1 Huth EJ (1986) Irresponsible authorship and wasteful publication. *Ann Intern Med.* **104**: 257–9.

2 Smith R (2002) New *BMJ* policy on economic evaluation. *BMJ.* **325**: 1124.

■ Secondary publications

Most studies produce one, fat, juicy publication reporting the main findings – this is termed the **primary publication**. Virtually everything else is considered a secondary publication. The distinction is important because secondary publications should not appear before the primary one and should always reference it. To avoid data from the same study getting included more than once in meta-analyses, it is also good practice to include a trial registration number on all publications, so readers can tell when different papers refer to the same trial.

Secondary publications can include sub-group analyses, follow-up studies and **translations**. Publications that do not present original data, such as review articles, may also be considered secondary publications.

■ Second target journal

Always select a second target journal in case you get rejected by your first target. Try to select the second journal at the same time as the first because you will have all the relevant journal information to hand and you may not get another chance to discuss this face to face if you are planning only one or two **meetings (of the writing group)**. If you do not select a second journal at this stage you may delay resubmission by trying to gather opinions. It may also be more difficult to reach agreement when everybody is in a bad mood after the first rejection.

■ Selective publication

Something to avoid: this is the practice of publishing only those studies that favour your product or theory, or of publishing only those parts of a study that are positive. In the first case, it leads to **publication bias**, which can distort the literature and skew meta-analyses. In the second, it produces misleading papers. One remedy for under-publication is **trial registration**, which has been a requirement for papers submitted to journals edited by the **International Committee of Medical Journal Editors (ICMJE)** committee members since July 2005. If a journal suspects selective publication of results, it may request a copy of the protocol. Many journals reserve the right to do this, and a few (e.g. *JAMA*, *The Lancet* and **PLOS**) require protocols to be submitted routinely.

Even if your intentions are honourable, you will sometimes have to decide which findings to omit from a short paper. One solution to the problem of presenting a large dataset within a stringent word limit is to publish **supplementary material** on the journal's website. Another solution is to produce more than one paper, but you should avoid **salami slicing**.

■ Self-archiving

The practice of posting your work after publication onto an institutional or personal website. This is allowed by some journals – to check which ones, you can use the **SHERPA/RoMEO** website.

■ SHERPA/FACT

This is a tool to enable researchers to check whether journals comply with UK funders' requirements for **Open Access** publication. You simply enter the name of the funder (e.g. Wellcome Trust) and the name of the journal. Unfortunately, it only works for UK funders.

www.sherpa.ac.uk/fact/index.php

■ SHERPA/JULIET

This website lists research funders' **Open Access** policies. It might be handy if you can't find your grant contract. It goes without saying that publication strategies should always comply with funders' requirements and, increasingly, many public funders (such as the UK Medical Research Council and the US National Institutes for Health) require researchers to publish their findings in an Open Access venue. The website's odd name arose because it is a companion to the RoMEO website and was developed by SHERPA (which stands for Securing a Hybrid Environment for Research Preservation and Access).

www.sherpa.ac.uk/juliet/index.php

■ SHERPA/RoMEO

Don't be put off by the odd name of this website; it is a fantastically useful resource for checking publishers' copyright and **self-archiving** policies (i.e. what you are allowed to do with your article after publication). In case you were wondering, RoMEO stands for Rights Meta-data for Open Archiving and it was developed by SHERPA (which stands for Securing a Hybrid Environment for Research Preservation and Access). Inevitably, it has a partner website, called **SHERPA/ JULIET**.

www.sherpa.ac.uk/romeo/

■ Short reports

In the olden days of ink and dead trees, parsimonious editors guarded their precious pages fiercely and encouraged short publications. This meant that short reports or research letters generally had higher acceptance rates than full-length articles. Now in the magical era of electronic publishing, the rules have changed. Some journals publish long web versions and shorter printed ones (*see* **ELPS**) so the truly short report may be on the verge of extinction. However, some old-fashioned journals whose print and web versions are identical may still include different formats and they are worth considering.

■ Short title; *see running title*

■ Slides

Slides are often used to illustrate **oral presentations** at meetings, but organisers rarely provide guidance about how to prepare them. If you do not have much experience of giving talks at conferences, or if the prospect worries you, consult friendly colleagues and/or books.

You should not give copies of your slides to journalists since this could lead to extensive reporting which might jeopardise full publication in a journal. However, you may provide your abstract since this is considered to be in the public domain. Although journals may permit webcasts from conferences, they may be less happy if a company or institution posts slides on its website before publication, so it is best to avoid this.

When working with co-authors or sponsors, ensure there is enough time for everybody to comment on the presentation. You will probably be allowed to talk for only about 10 minutes, so it is crucial to focus on your **key message** and decide what you are going to leave out. Unlike papers, graphs are often better than complex tables at conveying messages on slides.

Fraser J and Cave R (2004) *Presenting in Biomedicine: 500 tips for success.* Radcliffe Medical Press, Oxford.

Hall GM (ed.) (2001) *How to Present at Meetings.* BMJ Books, London.

■ Social media

Publishers, journal editors and some authors have been quick to embrace the social media such as Twitter and Facebook that sprung up around 2004–2006. There are even specialist sites designed to help scientists share their publications (e.g. ResearchGate) or discuss other people's publications (e.g. PubPeer), and metrics to capture social media activity (e.g. Altmetric). Advocates will tell you that promoting your publication via these routes can increase usage, while ignoring the circularity of the argument that mentioning something on Twitter increases the number of times that something gets mentioned on Twitter. It's early days, but there is some evidence that active promotion via social media generates downloads but it's hard to tell if it increases citations, so your view on this probably depends on which you regard as the most important measure of an article's use or impact. Pharmaceutical companies also need to be wary of marketing regulations and whether use of social media constitutes direct-to-consumer advertising, which is banned in many regions and controlled in others.

Even if you don't actively promote your own publications, should you join in discussions about them via social media? Again, it probably depends on whether you are a fan or foe of social media and, if you are a company, ensuring you remain compliant with relevant regulations.

On a point of peer-review etiquette, I once asked a journal editor who is active on social media whether it was acceptable to Tweet the fact that a manuscript had been submitted to a journal. Her advice was that it was fine to mention that the manuscript had been submitted but that we should not name the journal as this might cause confusion if it was rejected and ended up being published elsewhere and also that it might appear to be putting pressure on the journal to accept the article. It is obviously vital to keep all authors informed of the status of a submission, and you may need to inform a few other people such as the sponsor, but I agreed that it probably isn't helpful to broadcast a specific submission to the world – you should probably restrain your Tweets until the glorious moment of publication. Although accepted articles may be cited as being 'in press', watch out for journal **embargoes**, for example *JAMA*'s instructions state 'all information regarding the content and publication date of accepted manuscripts is strictly confidential' – so they don't want you Tweeting anything about it until it is published.

■ Sponsor, role of

Some journals require details about the exact role of the sponsor or funder in the research and publication process. For example, *The Lancet* requires information about the role, if any, of the sponsor in the study design; collection, analysis and interpretation of data; writing the report; and the decision to submit the paper for publication to be included under a subheading 'Role of the funding source' at the end of the methods section. **Good Publication Practice** (GPP3) also recommends that 'The role (if any) of the sponsor (e.g. funding of the study, its publication, or writing support; involvement in the design of the study or the collection, analysis, or interpretation of the data; or review of the manuscript) should always be clearly disclosed'.

■ Strategy

This term comes from the Greek word for army (*stratos*) and the verb to lead (*ago*). Although the mental image of warfare is perhaps unfortunate, it does remind us that lots of people are usually involved in publications, and that good leadership and communication are vital. However, unlike an army, there is rarely a single leader who can bark orders at the others and demand undying loyalty. A successful leader in terms of publications is someone who can guide the group with sound knowledge and facilitate decision making.

In both warfare and publications, it is important to have clear objectives and to ensure that these are shared by all members of the group (*see* **expectations** for more about this). A good strategy therefore starts with a clear agreement on what you want to achieve, for example presentations at international anaesthetics meetings in autumn 2017 and a full paper published in a respected, peer-reviewed anaesthetics journal by summer 2018. Once you have agreed the objective you can move on to your tactics, or plan (*see* Chapter 2 'Developing a publication plan for a multicentre study', pp. 7–11). This will involve choice of target meetings and journal, sorting out **authorship** and agreeing a detailed timetable for who does what.

If you are planning several publications from one piece of research (e.g. a couple of abstracts, a main paper and a secondary publication) it is important to plan them together to ensure a coherent strategy.

■ STROBE

Guidelines for Strengthening the Reporting of OBservational studies in Epidemiology which have been endorsed by many journals. Like **CONSORT**, these guidelines include a checklist, which you need to include when submitting to some journals. However, as the guidelines are more recent than CONSORT, not so many journals insist on this, but it certainly won't do any harm to use it.

www.strobe-statement.org

■ Style

If you are fanatical about writing style, and consider your own to be matchless, you should limit your writing to single-author works, which, these days, usually means editorials, reviews and books. Most research involves collaboration, and, while papers should not be written by committee, they should represent a team effort, which means that strong personal styles are out of place. The writer's style may be further compromised by the journal's **house style**, which is non-negotiable.

If you are preparing a research paper, and particularly if several people are drafting different sections, you should aim for a neutral style. This does not mean that the paper has to be wordy, jargon-ridden or boring, merely that you should curb any tendency to florid prose or personal idiosyncrasies. Once the fragments have been assembled and everybody has agreed on the content it is a good idea for one person to go through the whole paper to make the style as consistent as possible. Inconsistent style (as well as annoying readers) may, even if it has an innocent explanation, suggest **plagiarism** to eagle-eyed and suspicious editors.

If you find the mere thought of writing terrifying, and consider discussions of style to be more appropriate to literature classes or book clubs, take a recent issue of your **target journal** and read three or four papers describing broadly similar research to yours. This should give you a taste of the kind of style the journal prefers. If you cannot find papers describing research broadly similar to yours, you may have selected the wrong journal (in which case, read the section on **journal choice** again). Do not copy chunks of other papers, or try to follow their style too slavishly, but, if you are unsure how much detail to include, or get stuck trying to phrase something, it may help to re-read these papers when you are writing.

Your submission does not need to look exactly like the final journal page – this is the job of the technical editor and typesetter (*see* **house style**). However, you need to follow the instructions and ensure major features are correct, in particular the style for references. Submitting a paper styled for another journal creates a poor impression of carelessness or suspicions that it has already been rejected by another journal.

If you want to improve your writing style read:

Strunk W and White EB (1999) *The Elements of Style* (4e). Pearson/Longman. Also available at www.bartleby.com/141/.

■ Sub-editing; *see* technical editing

■ Submission fees

Nearly all journals that levy an **article processing charge** for publication require payment only after acceptance. However, a few journals charge a submission fee. For example, *Blood* charges 'a nonrefundable fee of $50' on submission of regular articles and brief reports (but not for review articles or letters to the editor). Similarly, the *Singapore Medical Journal* charges an 'administrative fee' unless you are a member of the Singapore Medical Association. If you have researched **target journals** carefully and believe such journals are right for your research, paying a nominal fee, while a slight hassle, should not put you off. However, beware any journal that asks for payment of larger sums on submission (rather than after acceptance) as it is possibly a sign that they are **predatory journals**.

■ Submission letter; *see* cover letter / covering letter

■ Subscription journals

This term is used to describe the traditional business model by which publishers fund journals by getting readers (or libraries) to pay a subscription to receive a copy or read the journal online. This distinguishes them from **Open Access** journals, which are free to read but usually charge authors an **article processing charge**. From an authors' point of view, the good thing about subscription journals is that they won't charge you to publish, but the bad thing about them is that they often have high rejection rates (because readers value selectivity) and, obviously, your article will only be available to readers who can afford to subscribe (or who work at an institution that can afford to subscribe). Some journals offer a **hybrid** model, allowing authors to make their article Open Access, if they pay an **article processing charge**, but charging readers a subscription to read other articles.

■ Sunshine Act

This innocent sounding piece of US legislation may have unintended consequences for company-sponsored publications. The Physician Payments Sunshine Act of 2010 was designed to increase transparency about payments from drug companies (and other commercial organisations) to American doctors. It requires companies to submit information about all transactions of over $10 with US doctors to a public website (www.cms.gov/openpayments/). The trouble, from the publication viewpoint, is that the information is supposed to include benefits in kind (termed 'transfers of value') as well as hard cash, but such benefits have not been clearly defined. So, if a company offers to pay a medical writer to help develop a publication from one of its studies, it is not clear if this could be viewed as a benefit to the authors under the terms of the Act. And, if it is a benefit, how should the value be divided among the authors? Some doctors consider that any payment from a drug company represents a conflict of interest and should be avoided, although they may be willing to take part in company-sponsored research, where funding usually goes to the department or institution rather than directly into the investigators' pockets. Such investigators may be unwilling to accept support from a professional medical writer if this would show up as a 'transfer of value' from a drug company on the public database. As the database is in its early days (it went public in September 2014), and the details of the legislation have yet to be worked out, companies appear to be using a variety of interpretations. Some companies argue that providing a medical writer to work on a publication benefits the company, rather than the investigator/author, and therefore need not be declared, but others disagree. Among companies that have decided to declare such transactions, there is no consensus about how this is done, for instance how the 'value' is divided between authors. These important aspects may be resolved in the coming years, so I can only advise you to stay alert. One source of information is the International Society for Medical Publication Professionals resource page: www.ismpp.org/sunshine-act-resources.

Sunshine Act legislation might also affect companies' largesse with reprints, since handing these to doctors is considered to be a transfer of value.

For discussions about reprints see:

www.policymed.com/2014/03/physician-payments-sunshine-act-best-practices-for-journal-reprint-valuation-physician-owners-and-recruits-pre-disclosures.html

www.cohealthcom.org/category/sunshine-act-2/

Before Europeans start feeling smug that these problems only beset our friends in the USA, they should be aware that similar legislation is (as of 2015) being proposed or initiated in several European countries. Australia has had a similar database since 2007 but as it only relates to industry-sponsored events it doesn't affect publications.

■ Supplementary material

Some journals publish short versions in the paper edition but permit (or even encourage) longer versions, or the provision of supplementary material, on their website. *The BMJ* refers to this principle as Electronic Long, Paper Short (or **ELPS**). If you have a very rich dataset, or information in a format unsuitable for print, such as extensive colour images, video clips or massive tables, you should check for this facility when choosing your target journal.

Check what formats the journal can accept, and at what stage. For example, you may not be able to submit video clips at the initial reviewing stage, but you should mention that they are available in your covering letter. Whenever possible, try to stick to word limits, and make it clear which material you would be prepared to consider supplementary to the print version (i.e. which may appear only on the website).

If you want to cite supplementary information, give the precise web address and the date you accessed it. Some journals assign special identifiers to electronic material or link electronic components to the paper version using the **DOI (Digital Object Identifier) system**.

■ Supplements

Some journals publish supplements, which are funded by a sponsor and usually cover a specific theme or present the proceedings of a meeting. Such sponsored supplements can be useful vehicles for publishing articles that might be of insufficient interest to be published in the parent journal. However, most journals will not accept papers that are of lower quality than those they normally publish. This was clearly not always the case, since a 1994 study showed that many readers' scepticism about material published in supplements was well founded.[1]

Most journals now state that supplements undergo similar peer review to the parent journal. However, this review is probably directed more to the scientific merit of the articles than to whether they are of interest to readers. Supplements have traditionally been used to repackage or collate several studies, for example to bring together preclinical research about a new drug. This can help readers who might not have access to the original work published in obscure journals. However, a supplement should not be viewed as a licence to create **redundant publication**, and secondary papers should clearly reference their primary sources.

If a supplement is used to present the proceedings of a meeting, you need to ensure that all presenters are happy for their work to appear in this form. There is no rule that new data should not be published in supplements, but this will preclude publication in another journal and may not be the author's first choice. References to supplements usually include the supplement number and may use a different page numbering system from the parent journal (e.g. Vol. 14 (Suppl. 1): S17–32), making it clear to sharp-eyed readers that they did not appear in the main journal. Given the slightly tarnished reputation of supplements, it is usually a better strategy to publish primary papers elsewhere.

Some journals insist that supplements are edited by somebody from outside the sponsoring organisation (although this does not preclude professional writing assistance).

If you are considering a supplement, first check that your target journal actually produces these, and then contact the journal to discover how it handles them. You will need to find out how material is reviewed (and how long this will take), what the costs are and if there are any special requirements, such as having an independent editor.

1 Rochon P, Gurwitz JH, Cheung CM *et al.* (1994) Evaluating the quality of articles published in journal supplements compared with the quality of those published in the parent journal. *JAMA.* **272**: 108–13.

T

■ Tables

Deciding which data are best presented in tables is an important aspect of planning a paper. Most journals do not allow data to be repeated in text, tables and **figures**, so you need to choose the best format. Remember that a table should normally include at least two columns of figures – most journals will not accept tables with only one column of data, as this can easily be expressed as a list (which takes up less space). However, single-column tables are acceptable for posters. Some congresses allow small tables in abstracts, and this can be a good way to present results, but check the congress requirements since many do not.

You should start planning the tables when the **data analysis plan** is being developed to ensure that the statistical report provides the information you need for the publication.

When preparing a paper, keep tables separate from the text, at the end of the paper. Even if they look inelegant and spill on to more than one page, manuscript tables should always be double-spaced. For electronic submissions it is important to use the table function or tabs on your word processing software – do not separate columns using simple word spacing as the data are likely to get garbled. Most journal tables do not include vertical lines to separate columns, so you should avoid using these. Even if you have submitted a carefully prepared electronic version of your manuscript, pay particular attention to tables in the proofs, as numbers often get displaced when word-processed tables are converted for page layout. The best way to proofread a complex table is to ask a colleague to read out the numbers from the original version while you check the proof.

For more information about tables try Chapter 14 in:

Huth EJ (1999) *Writing and Publishing in Medicine* (3e). Williams & Wilkins, Baltimore.

■ Target audience

Identifying your readers is an important step in planning any publication since it should influence your choice of meeting or journal and the way in which you present the findings. To identify your target audience, think hard about who might actually be interested in your findings rather than who you think ought to be interested. (This is sometimes called the 'Who cares?' test.) Consider not only who your ideal readers are (e.g. haematologists) but where they work (e.g. Europe) and how advanced they are in their specialty (e.g. consultants).

Identifying the target audience for each publication is not only a key part of the publication strategy, but also helps to focus the writing and determine the **key message**. If the authors are not members of the target audience (e.g. specialists writing for generalists) try to include somebody from the target audience in your **internal review**.

■ Target journal

Agree on the journal to which you will submit your paper (i.e. your target) as early as possible. Writing a paper before you have defined your target journal can be a waste of time because it indicates that you have not really considered your **target audience** and it also means you will have to go back and check requirements for length, style and **formatting**. *See also* **journal choice** for more details.

■ Technical editing

This may be considered the final stage of the peer-review process (unless one counts **post-publication comments**). Technical editing (also called copy editing or sub-editing) involves checking the submission carefully, correcting or improving the language and putting it into the journal's **house style**. Major journals usually employ (or hire) professional copy editors. Although such copy editors lack specialist qualifications most are skilled at spotting inconsistencies and errors that expert reviewers and authors fail to notice. In some smaller journals, the job of technical editing falls to the editor or members of the **editorial board**.

The amount of technical editing that your paper undergoes will depend on the journal. Some (e.g. the '**Big Five**' and many traditional specialty journals) invest heavily in this; others (mostly the newer, electronic journals) do hardly any at all. You can judge the degree of technical editing practised by a journal by perusing back issues. If all articles not only have a clear house style in terms of spelling (e.g. US or UK), abbreviations and layout, but also have a certain uniformity of prose style, they are likely to have been heavily edited. If you are submitting to a journal that does minimal copy editing you might choose to get a professional copy editor, or a colleague with a talent for this sort of thing, to check your final version and proofs.

If your work has been heavily edited there is little you can (or should) do about this, unless the editing has introduced ambiguity or changed your meaning, in which case you should politely point this out and correct the problem on the proofs. However, if the copy editor changes your meaning, resist the urge simply to change the text back to the original, since, if the copy editor did not understand you, there is a good chance that some readers will have the same problem, so it makes sense to try to find an alternative wording.

There is some evidence that technical editing improves the readability of papers.[1] However, many people who enjoy writing and have developed a strong personal style dislike having that **style** diluted and their 'voice' removed.

1 Wager E and Middleton P (2002) Effects of technical editing in biomedical journals: a systematic review. *JAMA*. **287**: 2821–4.

■ Text recycling

This term is used to describe authors' reuse of their own words, usually without mentioning the source or the fact that the text has appeared in previous publications. However, there is no precise definition of text recycling or clear guidance about when it constitutes a problem and may be considered as **redundant publication**. Guidelines produced by some editors from **BioMed Central** and promoted by the **Committee on Publication Ethics**[1] stress that judgement is required (in other words, it is up to the editor to decide). Authors and publication planners preparing multiple publications from a single trial or dataset, or even just a few publications on similar topics, need to be aware of how much text recycling journals will tolerate and the fact that text-matching software is widely used and is highly sensitive even to small amounts of repetition. If in doubt, check that previous publications are cited and consider attaching any overlapping or related publications as supplementary files when you submit a new work so the journal can see you are not trying to hide anything and the editor can decide if any repetition is justified.

1 http://publicationethics.org/text-recycling-guidelines

■ The Publication Plan; *see* Publication Plan, The

■ 'Throwaways'; *see freebies*

■ Timing

So many factors can affect the timing of a publication that it is impossible to summarise in a short entry. Consult Chapter 3 'How long will it take?' (pp. 13–17) for more details but remember that best case scenarios are rare occurrences, humans are fallible, most people involved in developing publications have chronically over-filled diaries, and we all know what happens to the 'best laid plans of mice and men …', although, I have to admit that I have never yet come across a mouse who was planning to publish any research.

■ Title
■ Papers and abstracts

Take care composing the title of your publications, since a good title can attract readers, while a poor one may be the only section they read. Check the requirements of your target meeting or journal. Conferences sometimes limit the length of abstract titles, while some journals specify what you should, or should not, include. In general, you should avoid abbreviations, unless they are universally understood (such as DNA). You should also avoid using drug trade names, since many journals forbid their use in the title, and brand names often differ from country to country, so it is best to use the generic name. Use of the trade name in the title may also give your publication an unduly commercial feel and prejudice some reviewers and readers.

Creating a good title is a balancing act between including all the pertinent information and keeping it short. In your efforts to restrict the number of words avoid 'noun strings' which can be hard to read. A noun string occurs when too many nouns act as adjectives, for example: 'Oral iron supplementation induced intestinal oxidative stress'. Although it takes a few more words, it is clearer to write: 'Intestinal oxidative stress induced by oral iron supplementation'.

Aim to begin with important words, which will interest the reader, and put details such as the trial design at the end (otherwise most titles will begin 'A randomised, controlled study of …'). Check your target journal for its **house style** regarding punctuation or subtitles (e.g. *The BMJ* has a fondness for colons, so you will often see the format 'X versus Y in dread disease: a randomised controlled trial'). Including details of the trial design in the title may increase your chance of the publication being correctly indexed and therefore retrieved by researchers.

While brand names should be avoided, trial names can be useful since they identify related publications. However, ingenious acronyms for trials have become so fashionable that there is a slight risk that you will pick an acronym already used by another study, and thus cause confusion. For this reason use of a less exciting

trial identifier, such as a protocol number or **trial registration** number, may be better.

Some journals allow declarative (or informative) titles, which describe your results, for example: 'Wunderdrug improves glycaemic control in type II diabetes'. However, many journals permit only descriptive (or indicative) titles which describe the study but not the results, for example 'Glycaemic control in type II diabetes: a randomised, placebo-controlled trial of Wunderdrug'.

When writing the title for an **abstract**, remember you will have to use the same title if you present as a **poster**, so think about how it looks and whether it will stand out from the crowd. Questions and short titles may be more effective at grabbing attention than the detailed titles often used for journal articles.

Good titles arouse potential readers' curiosity without being opaque or baffling. You can be more creative with titles for editorials and reviews than for trial reports, but remember that your audience may not share a common culture, so references to your favourite pop song, television series or children's book may confuse rather than enlighten many readers. Titles that pose a question or conjure up a strong mental image can grab readers' attention – I once entitled a rather dull essay on regulations governing doctors' relations with drug companies, 'How to dance with porcupines', and was pleasantly surprised how much positive feedback I got.

■ Journals

Do not be fooled by journal titles: they are not always a good indication of a journal's scope or nature. Some journals retain titles that have little bearing on their current contents – for example, the *Philosophical Transactions of the Royal Society (B)* is a respected biology journal dating from the 17th century when natural history was called philosophy. Even recent journals may have undergone a change in emphasis so that their title no longer reflects their content – for example, the *Journal of Experimental Medicine* is about immunology. Others have such mundane titles that it is impossible to guess what will interest them. When assessing possible **target journals** look at three to six of the most recent issues to determine the scope, accepted formats, **hot topics**, length of articles, etc. If you don't have access to the journal, check the website for contents lists or a sample issue. If that fails, contact the publisher who will usually be prepared to supply a sample copy.

■ Title page

Check the journal's requirements and gather all the information you need for the title page of your submission as early as possible. Get authors to check their details on the first draft they see and do not be tempted to leave this section until just before submission (when you can be sure that at least one author will be uncontactable and you will waste valuable time chasing irritating details).

All journals will require the authors' names (*see* **names** for how to present these), their **affiliation** (now and when they did the work) and full contact details for the corresponding author (including fax and e-mail). Many US journals also require authors' highest degrees.

■ Translations

To make your research accessible to a wide audience you might consider presentations at local meetings and publications in several languages. Local language journals have an important role in reaching clinicians but are often considered less prestigious (and have lower **impact factors**) than English language journals. Before considering a translation, always check the copyright status and whether you need permission from the original publisher. Some journals will consider translations of published papers but these must reference the original paper and be faithful to the source (e.g. they should not contain new material). An alternative (and sometimes quicker) solution is to ask the original journal for reprint translations. Major publishers are often happy to provide these (for a fee). If you prepare a new version for a second audience (e.g. with emphasis on local findings) take care that this does not constitute **redundant publication**.

■ Trial identifier

Some trials generate several publications. These can be legitimate, for example a couple of abstracts, a primary paper and a follow-up report or secondary analysis, but they may represent **redundant publication** and contribute to **publication bias**. One simple solution for preventing confusion is to include a trial identifier on all publications. Trial identifiers allow readers to see whether publications are linked (e.g. which full reports relate to previous abstracts or other publications) and remove the risk of inadvertently double-counting trials in meta-analysis. **Good Publication Practice (GPP)** recommends that trial identifiers should be included on all publications (including abstracts).

A trial identifier may simply be the sponsor's protocol number, or may be linked with inclusion in a public trial register. Since July 2005 members of the **International Committee of Medical Journal Editors (ICMJE)** have required **trial registration** as a condition for publication in their journals and GPP3 also supports this.

So far, conference organisers have not come out in support of trial identifiers, and it may be difficult to squeeze this information on to an abstract if space is limited. One possible solution is to refer to the trial name in the title or include a group name in the author list (e.g. Bloggs & Cloggs on behalf of the AQ153 Study Group). However, not all conference websites permit this. Another option is to include the trial identifier within the funding acknowledgement (e.g. this study was funded by the Wunderdrug Corporation, trial registration number ZZ123).

Wager E (2004) The need for trial identifiers. *Curr Med Res Opin.* **20**: 203–6.

■ Trial registration

Groups that prepare systematic reviews, such as the Cochrane Collaboration, have long argued that details of all trials should be prospectively entered on to a register so that researchers, and potential participants, can see what trials are taking place or have been completed. In this way, they argue, **publication bias** caused by non-publication of unfavourable findings will be prevented. Various trial registers have been established but until recently they were largely voluntary and did not have much to do with publications. However, in September 2004, the members of the **International Committee of Medical Journal Editors (ICMJE)** announced that trial registration would be a requirement for publication in their journals from July 2005. (For a list of the ICMJE members, *see* **International Committee of Medical Journal Editors**.) Since then, many other journals have followed the ICMJE's lead in making prospective registration a requirement (i.e. trials must be registered when they start and the registration number must be stated in all publications). **Good Publication Practice** (GPP3) also supports trial registration and recommends that any unregistered studies should be 'declared as such, and the reason for nonregistration should be provided'.

De Angelis C, Drazen JM, Frizelle FA *et al.* (2004) Clinical trial registration: a statement from the International Committee of Medical Journal Editors. *Lancet.* **364**: 911–12.

U

■ 'Uniform requirements'; *see* International Committee of Medical Journal Editors (ICMJE)

■ Unpublished data (references to)

If you want to refer to unpublished data you need to be aware of some general rules and of individual journal restrictions on this (since they vary).

Once a paper has been accepted for publication it can be cited as being 'in press'. Such a reference looks the same as any other, with a full list of authors, title and journal details, and, where possible, the expected year of publication, but the journal volume and page numbers are simply replaced by the words 'in press'. Only papers that have been accepted (in full) may be cited as 'in press'. A conditional acceptance (i.e. a statement that the journal will reconsider the paper or might publish if the reviewers' comments can be addressed) does *not* mean the paper is 'in press' since it is possible that the journal will not publish it. Some journals therefore require a copy of the acceptance letter to establish that an article is truly 'in press' and that the author is not being over-optimistic.

Submitting work to a journal or meeting does *not* equate to it being 'in press'. This may be frustrating, but consider it from the reader's viewpoint. If a reference lists something as, for example, 'submitted to *The Lancet*' there is a strong chance (>90%) that the paper will be rejected, and will therefore not appear in *The Lancet*. Moreover, when the paper is finally accepted, or sent to another journal, the title (and possibly even the author list) may have changed, so it may be difficult for the reader to locate the reference.

Most journals allow citation of published abstracts and associated presentations at meetings, but some, for example *Circulation*, do not. Such citations usually include the name of the meeting, its location and date, as well as the abstract title and authors' names. If the abstract also appears in a journal you should include its title since readers are more likely to have access to journals than to conference proceedings. For example, abstracts presented at the American Society of Hematology appear in a special edition of the journal *Blood*. Some journals (e.g. *Annals of Internal Medicine*) will only accept references published in journals.

If your **target journal** does not permit you to cite an abstract or presentation you may have to include it as a **personal communication** giving brief details in the text, but nothing in the reference list.

ClinicalTrials.gov gives guidance on how to cite studies in this database. See www.nlm.nih.gov/services/ctcite/html.

V

 Vancouver Group

Another name for the **International Committee of Medical Journal Editors (ICJME)** – because they first met in Vancouver.

 Verbal branding

'Verbal branding' is a marketing term, but, even if you think your publication has nothing to do with marketing, read on, because you need to understand it if you work with drug companies, and you might even find the concept helpful in non-commercial research. Verbal branding simply means the careful and consistent choice of words.

While it usually applies to a pharmaceutical product, verbal branding can be used to deliver any message consistently and effectively. Good communicators probably use verbal branding instinctively by choosing powerful phrases to get their message across.

Some companies develop preferred terms and phrases for describing their products and their competitors. Preferred language may even extend to the drug's indications, and companies have sometimes been accused of creating or promoting new diseases. However, some new terms are more precise or less stigmatising than traditional ones, so they should not all be dismissed as marketing gimmicks. The company's usual aim is to harmonise product descriptions used in promotional material and in the scientific literature so that publications reinforce marketing messages and strengthen the brand image.

The words used to describe mental illness are a good example of the power of language. Disparaging and insensitive terms such as 'spastic' and 'mentally deficient' have now been replaced by 'cerebral palsy' and 'learning disability'. Similarly, powerful painkillers tend to be called opioids rather than narcotics, because of associations with drug abuse. On the subject of drugs, have you ever noticed how critical articles tend to refer to drug companies, while the firms refer to themselves as the pharmaceutical industry?

If you think that verbal branding will lead to repetitive writing, I can only refer you to Fowler's splendid tirade against what he calls 'elegant variation' (i.e. the mistake of believing you must use different words if you mention something more than once):[1]

> It is the second-rate writers, those intent rather on expressing themselves prettily than on conveying their meaning clearly, and still more those whose notions of style are based on a few misleading rules of thumb, that are chiefly open to the allurements of elegant variation. … The fatal influence is the advice given to young writers never to use the same word twice in a sentence – or within 20 lines or other limit.

Remember that, while preferred spellings and formats can be used on internal documents and marketing material, peer-reviewed journals impose their own **house style** on papers, so these details may be changed in the final publication. Also, most journals insist that generic product names should be used in papers, and restrict the use of trade names, which can usually be mentioned only once, in the methods section, and often may not be used in titles. When preparing articles for submission to peer-review journals it is therefore important to follow journal guidelines and to be aware that the journal will impose its house style on the published version.

1 Fowler HW (1965) *A Dictionary of Modern English Usage* (2e). Oxford University Press, Oxford.

■ Veto

Research sponsors, be they commercial companies, charities or public institutions, should not have the right to veto a publication. Researchers should check their **contract** or **publication agreement** carefully to ensure they are free to publish their findings.

Differences of opinion may arise between sponsors and investigators, and also between co-authors. The best way to avoid protracted negotiations from delaying the publication schedule is to involve all interested parties in the earliest stages of planning. Ideally, everybody should meet to discuss the findings and agree the publication strategy. If a meeting is not possible, all **key players** should be given the opportunity to comment on the plan. If everybody agrees on the **outline** for each publication this will greatly reduce the risk of differences in interpretation scuppering the schedule.

Many contracts allow sponsors the right to delay a publication, usually to protect intellectual property (e.g. if a patent is being filed). Many sponsors also expect to be given the opportunity to review a publication before it is submitted. When planning a publication schedule you need to build this time (often 30 days, but sometimes 60 or even 90) into the plan. When planning to submit an abstract it is especially important to allow time for review by colleagues, institutional bosses and the sponsor.

As an individual contributor to a study, if you disagree strongly with the way in which the results are presented or interpreted your only weapons are your power of persuasion and reasoned argument. If agreement cannot be reached, you can withdraw your name from the list of authors, but you cannot veto a publication.

■ Vicious reviewers

A review of a paper should never contain disparaging remarks about the authors and should, in an ideal world, be courteous even if it is damning. If you receive a discourteous review you might mention this in your response to the journal but, especially if the reviewer recommends rejection, be careful not to sound peevish yourself and be sure to distinguish between the style and the substance.

See **zealots** for more discussion about consistently harsh reviewers. If you feel you have been the victim of an unduly harsh review, it may be worth appealing, but it is often best to try another journal.

W

◼ Waivers; *see* article processing charge

◼ WAME; *see* World Association of Medical Editors

◼ Web publication / institutional websites

Most medical journals regard posting on a **preprint** server, or on a personal or institutional website, to be equivalent to publication and you should therefore avoid doing this before your paper has been published. However, some journals, including those that make contents available only to subscribers, now permit or even encourage such posting *after* publication (this is sometimes called **Green Open Access**). Before posting (either before or after publication) you should therefore check with the journal or on **SHERPA/RoMEO**. Journals that operate an **Open Access** policy generally permit authors to post their own material, or to include a link to the journal website from their own. **BioMed Central** has recently launched Open Repository, a commercial service to help institutions administer publication archives. See www.biomedcentral.com for details.

Perhaps surprisingly, most journals do not consider a 'webcast' from a meeting to constitute prior publication.[1]

1 Kassirer JP (1999) Posting presentations at medical meetings on the internet. *N Engl J Med*. **340**: 803.

◼ Withdrawal

If you discover a serious problem with your work before publication, contact the journal or conference immediately and ask to withdraw it. Despite everybody's best efforts and expertise, mistakes do happen, and most editors will appreciate your honesty.

However, abstracts and papers should not be withdrawn simply because a company's policies or priorities have changed. Some conferences accept **placeholder abstracts** which describe the design of a study but not the results. It is not good practice to withdraw these if results turn out unfavourably to your product or theory. Companies and researchers should commit to publishing all their studies, otherwise they will be contributing to **publication bias**. However, if you submit an abstract in good faith and then do not have any meaningful results to present by the time of the meeting, for example because of delays in recruitment, withdrawal may be acceptable.

If a journal discovers that it has published a flawed or misleading paper (either because of a genuine error or because of scientific misconduct) it may retract the paper. The notice of retraction should appear in indexing systems that cover the journal. Although, in complex studies, contributors may take responsibility for only part of the research, all authors (or contributors) will be affected by such a retraction, so think hard before putting your name on a paper if you have any doubts about it. Similarly, it is not usually possible to withdraw your name from a paper once it has been published – although, if serious problems come to light after publication the journal might allow you to publish a letter or statement outlining your concerns.

■ World Association of Medical Editors (WAME)

This is the newest of the associations for medical editors, founded in 1995. Unlike the **Council of Science Editors (CSE)** and **European Association of Science Editors (EASE)** it is a virtual organisation, relying largely on electronic communication rather than meetings. Whereas CSE is predominantly North American and EASE is largely European, WAME is more global, with members in over 90 countries. WAME has developed a number of policy statements, which can be found at www.wame.org.

Members can also take part in an electronic discussion forum.

WAME has an ethics committee, which considers anonymised cases submitted by members and aims to provide expert opinion. This function is similar to that of the **Committee on Publication Ethics (COPE)**, although it is more international and does not involve any face-to-face meetings.

■ World Medical Association (WMA)

Best known for issuing the Declaration of Helsinki, which sets out doctors' ethical responsibilities when doing research. The latest version (issued in 2013) states 'Negative and inconclusive as well as positive results must be published' and 'Researchers have a duty to make publicly available the results of their research on human subjects and are accountable for the completeness and accuracy of their reports'.

For more details go to www.wma.net.

Not to be confused with WAME (the **World Association of Medical Editors**).

■ Writing

If you started reading this book from 'A' and have reached 'W' expecting information about how to write scientific articles, prepare to be dismayed. Developing skill in writing will undoubtedly increase your chances of acceptance, but this is a book about publication strategy, and many fine books on writing have already been published. Sorry to disappoint you, but I recommend you go out and buy:

Albert T (2000) *The A–Z of Medical Writing*. BMJ Books, London.

Albert T (2000) *Winning the Publications Game* (2e). Radcliffe Medical Press, Oxford.

Fraser J (1997) *How to Publish in Biomedicine: 500 tips for success*. Radcliffe Medical Press, Oxford.

Goodman NW, Edwards MB and Langdon-Neuner E (2014) *Medical Writing: a prescription for clarity* (4e). Cambridge University Press, Cambridge.

Hall G (ed.) (2012) *How to Write a Paper* (5e). Wiley-Blackwell, Oxford.

Lang TA (2009) *How to Write, Publish and Present in the Health Sciences: a guide for physicians and laboratory researchers*. American College of Physicians, Philadelphia.

Strunk W and White EB (1999) *The Elements of Style* (4e). Pearson/Longman. Also available at www.bartleby.com/141/.

■ Writing group

If one considers the first criterion for **authorship** recommended by the **International Committee of Medical Journal Editors (ICMJE)** (i.e. involvement in study design, or data analysis and interpretation, or data acquisition) it quickly becomes apparent that, in all but the smallest clinical trials, more people could potentially qualify as authors than can practically be included. However, the ICMJE recommendations go on to say that authors must also be involved in preparing or reviewing the manuscript. The distinction between potential authors and actual ones therefore often depends on who is involved in developing the manuscript. It can therefore be helpful to designate a writing group at the start of a study.

If writing group members are identified early, study organisers can make sure that they have the opportunity to fulfil this role properly, e.g. by being given a chance to review and comment on the data and shape publications. Clear communication about how the writing group will function should also ensure that everybody has realistic expectations about who will be named as an author, and who is expected to do what.

There are no rules, and until now little published guidance, about the ideal size for writing groups. To some extent, this will depend on the scale of the trial and the number of people involved in study design and data interpretation. However, it is possible for a small coordinating group to be responsible for a trial involving many investigators (and therefore patients), so sheer numbers can be misleading.

Similarly, a relatively small trial (in terms of patients) involving complex, multidisciplinary assessment might merit a longer list of authors to ensure that all aspects are properly represented.

The ICMJE criteria also state that authors should be prepared to take public responsibility for at least some aspect of the research. This is a useful rule in deciding who qualifies to join the writing group. Hard work alone does not justify authorship, and unless someone could stand up in public and answer questions about the rationale behind the study design, or what the results really mean, then they probably do not qualify as an author.

This means that the writing group may include members who do not qualify as authors – for example a professional medical writer, or an author's editor, brought in at a relatively late stage to coordinate the process of developing publications.

Anybody who made substantial contributions to the study design and interpretation of the data obviously qualifies for authorship and should automatically be included in the writing group. However, investigators who recruited large numbers of patients (i.e. were involved in acquiring the data) will only qualify if given the opportunity to be involved in the publication. The study organisers will therefore have to decide how many people to involve. This is sometimes decided by a simple (and therefore arbitrary) formula, such as inviting the top three recruiters, or the top recruiter from each country. So long as these people are given a chance to be actively involved in developing the manuscript they will fulfil authorship criteria but, to avoid unrealistic expectations and disappointment at the end of the study, it is important to set out the rules from the start. **Good Publication Practice** (GPP3) notes that 'many [people] may be involved in the design and execution of clinical trials' and therefore 'it is not feasible to offer the opportunity of authorship to all of them. Priority should be given to the key contributors who have the necessary background to analyze or interpret the findings'.

In purely practical terms, so long as it includes members with sufficient expertise, the smaller the writing group, the faster the publication process. The more people who are involved in discussing, drafting and reviewing a manuscript, the longer it will take to finalise. However, the writing group needs to include sufficient people to do the work and to represent all aspects of the trial. Between three and six members is probably ideal for most studies. More than eight members (which may be necessary for large, complex trials) will inevitably slow down the process because more comments have to be taken into consideration and it will be slower to reach consensus. It is also harder to arrange face-to-face meetings for larger groups, and this may further delay the process (since a meeting is often the fastest and most efficient way to agree final wording, rather than endless rounds of e-mail comments or ear-bending telephone conferences, which also become unworkable with many participants).

However, keeping the group small should never be used as an excuse to exclude somebody who deserves **authorship**. The ICMJE guidelines clearly state that all those who qualify as authors should be included. The **Good Publication Practice (GPP)** guidelines also recommend that, whatever criteria are used to select authors, they should be applied consistently to external investigators and company employees in industry-sponsored studies. For more information about people who qualify as authors but are omitted, *see* **ghost authors**.

So, to summarise:

- start to think about the composition of the writing group early in the study
- communicate this decision, or the rules that will be applied, to everybody involved with the study
- ensure that writing group members have the opportunity to make a real contribution to developing the publication
- do not exclude anybody from the group who meets the authorship criteria
- but, if possible, keep the group to a reasonable size (three to six members is ideal).

X

■ Xenophobia (geographical bias)

Geographical bias (which has to appear under its slightly exaggerated and rather pompous form because I could not think of anything else that began with 'X') definitely exists to some degree, and a good strategy therefore needs to take it into consideration. At its mildest form, it simply means that North American journals prefer to publish North American studies, and the same holds true for other regions. This may have more to do with journal editors knowing what will interest their readers than a bias or prejudice against studies performed elsewhere, but sometimes a bit of the latter probably creeps in.

The former editor of *The Journal of the Norwegian Medical Association*, Magne Nylenna, and colleagues demonstrated one type of xenophobia rather neatly.[1] They sent a poor quality paper to 180 Scandinavian reviewers, either in English or in their native language. Reviewers who received the English version gave it higher ratings, on average, than those who received it in their native tongue. This suggests a bias against non-English language papers, although the effect was not significant when reviewers were sent a higher quality paper.

Another study by Egger *et al.* found that reports published in German were less likely to have statistically significant findings than those published in English.[2] This observation may have several causes, including the fact that English language journals tend to have wider readerships and higher **impact factors**, which may lead authors to send their 'better' results to international journals and publish less interesting findings in national journals.

When planning a publication strategy, it is important to identify your **target audience** and its location. People tend to be more interested about things that happen close to home, and there may be important geographic differences in the incidence or course of a disease, or the way in which it is treated. Defining your target readership will help focus your discussion on the most relevant, and therefore interesting, aspects.

1 Nylenna M, Riis P and Karlsson Y (1994) Multiple blinded reviews of the same two manuscripts. Effects of referee characteristics and publication language. *JAMA*. **272**: 149–51.

2 Egger M, Zellweger-Zähner T, Schneider M *et al.* (1997) Language bias in randomised controlled trials published in English and German. *Lancet*. **350**: 326–9.

Y

■ Young reviewers

Selecting reviewers is perhaps the most important role of a journal editor. Since most journals do not pay their reviewers, editors usually try to create a large database to spread the load and ensure good coverage in all subjects. The biggest names in a field will probably be in high demand from several journals (and already busy people). Furthermore, one study has shown that younger reviewers (aged <40) tend to produce the best reviews.[1]

1 Black N, van Rooyen S, Godlee F *et al.* (1998) What makes a good reviewer and a good review for a general medical journal? *JAMA*. **280**: 231–3.

Z

■ Zealots and assassins

An A–Z needs an entry for 'Z', and, fortunately, a study of peer reviewers in *Radiology* provides the answer.[1] This journal asks reviewers to rate papers from one (accept) to nine (reject). Siegelman set out to discover if some reviewers recommended rejection much more or less often than others and he called these two extremes assassins and zealots. Reassuringly, nearly 90% of the *Radiology* reviewers were neither assassins nor zealots, but gave ratings within ±1.5 standard deviations of the mean; about 5% fell into each of the intermediate categories of 'pushovers' who generally recommended acceptance (and gave ratings 1.5 standard deviations below the mean) and 'demoters' who generally recommended rejection (and gave ratings 1.5 standard deviations above the mean). About 1% of reviewers fell into each of the extreme categories of assassins or zealots. Having identified the reviewers from their average scores, Siegelman examined submissions that had been reviewed by pairs of reviewers from different categories (e.g. by an assassin and a mainstream reviewer) and showed that the reviewers gave consistently different ratings, suggesting that the categories were valid and had not arisen because some reviewers had, by chance, received either high or low quality submissions.

Siegelman suggests that editors might reduce unfairness in the peer-review process by weeding out the assassins and zealots from reviewer databases. *Radiology* uses a computerised database that allows editors to monitor reviewers' average scores and thus select a balance of reviewers (or at least ensure that no paper is reviewed only by assassins or zealots).

While it is always tempting to consider any reviewer who recommends rejecting your submission a biased assassin, you need to remember that, in most cases, the reviewer is only advising the editor, not providing the final judgement. If you receive wildly divergent reviews it might be worth appealing the decision, although this can be time-consuming and it may be better to seek another journal. If you think your paper has been the victim of an assassin, you could use Siegelman's study to support your argument and ask whether the journal monitors its reviewers' performance.

1 Siegelman SS (1991) Assassins and zealots: variations in peer review. Special report. *Radiology*. **178**: 637–42.

APPENDIX 1

Further reading

Albert T (2000) *The A–Z of Medical Writing*. BMJ Books, London.

Albert T (2000) *Winning the Publications Game* (2e). Radcliffe Medical Press, Oxford.

American Medical Association (2007) *AMA Manual of Style: a guide for authors and editors* (10e). JAMA/Oxford University Press, New York.

Council of Science Editors (CSE) (2014) *Scientific Style and Format: the CSE manual for authors, editors, and publishers* (8e). CSE/University of Chicago Press, Chicago.

Fraser J (1997) *How to Publish in Biomedicine: 500 tips for success*. Radcliffe Medical Press, Oxford.

Godlee F and Jefferson T (eds) (2003) *Peer Review in Health Sciences* (2e). BMJ Books, London.

Goodman NW, Edwards MB and Langdon-Neuer E (2014) *Medical Writing: a prescription for clarity* (4e). Cambridge University Press, Cambridge.

Hall GM (ed.) (2012) *How to Write a Paper* (5e). Wiley-Blackwell, Oxford.

Hudson Jones A and McLellan F (eds) (2000) *Ethical Issues in Biomedical Publication*. Johns Hopkins University Press, Baltimore.

Huth EJ (1999) *Writing and Publishing in Medicine* (3e). Williams & Wilkins, Baltimore.

Lang TA (2009) *How to Write, Publish, and Present in the Health Sciences: a guide for physicians and laboratory researchers*. American College of Physicians, Philadelphia.

Lang TA and Secic M (2006) *How to Report Statistics in Medicine: annotated guidelines for authors, editors, and reviewers* (2e). American College of Physicians, Philadelphia.

Smith R (2006) *The Trouble with Medical Journals*. Royal Society of Medicine Press, London.

Strunk W and White EB (1999) *The Elements of Style* (4e). Pearson/Longman. Also available at www.bartleby.com/141/.

Wager E, Godlee F and Jefferson T (2002) *How to Survive Peer Review*. BMJ Books, London.

Organisations

(*See also* entries in A to Z section, listed under full names, for more details.)

AMWA	American Medical Writers Association	www.amwa.org
COPE	Committee on Publication Ethics	www.publicationethics.org
CSE	Council of Science Editors	www.councilscienceeditors.org
EASE	European Association of Science Editors	www.ease.org.uk
EMWA	European Medical Writers Association	www.emwa.org
EQUATOR	EQUATOR Network (link to reporting guidelines)	www.equator-network.org
ICMJE	International Committee of Medical Journal Editors	www.icmje.org
ISMPP	International Society for Medical Publication Professionals	www.ismpp.org (website also includes Good Publication Practice [GPP3])
ISMTE	International Society for Managing and Technical Editors	www.ismte.org
PhRMA	Pharmaceutical Research and Manufacturers of America	www.phrma.org
WAME	World Association of Medical Editors	www.wame.org
WMA	World Medical Association	www.wma.net

Guidelines

AMWA Code of Ethics	www.amwa.org/amwa_ethics
Declaration of Helsinki	www.wma.net/ en/30publications/10policies/b3/ index.html
EMWA Guidelines on the Role of Medical Writers in Developing Peer-reviewed Publications	www.emwa.org/documents/about_ us/EMWAguidelines.pdf
Good Publication Practice (GPP3)	www.ismpp.org/gpp3
ICMJE Recommendations	www.icmje.org
ISMPP Code of Ethics	www.ismpp.org/code-of-ethics-a
PhRMA *Principles on Conduct of Clinical Trials and Communication of Trial Results*	www.phrma.org/sites/default/files/ pdf/042009_clinical_trial_principles_ final_0.pdf
The EQUATOR Network	www.equator-network.org has links to many reporting guidelines

APPENDIX 4

Principles of good publication practice for company-sponsored medical research (from GPP3)

1. The design and results of all clinical trials should be reported in a complete, accurate, balanced, transparent, and timely manner.
2. Reporting and publication processes should follow applicable laws (e.g. Food and Drug Administration Amendments Act of 2007) and guidelines (e.g. International Committee of Medical Journal Editors [ICMJE] recommendations and reporting guidelines found on the Enhancing the QUAlity and Transparency Of health Research [EQUATOR] Network).
3. Journal and congress requirements should be followed, especially ethical guidelines on originality and avoiding redundancy (i.e. duplicate publication).
4. Publication planning and development should be a collaboration among all persons involved (e.g. clinicians, statisticians, researchers, and publication professionals, including medical writers) and reflect the collaborative nature of research and the range of skills required to conduct, analyze, interpret, and report research findings.
5. The rights, roles, requirements, and responsibilities of all contributors (i.e. authors and any nonauthor contributors) should be confirmed in writing, ideally at the start of the research and, in all cases, before publication preparation begins.
6. All authors should have access to relevant aggregated study data and other information (e.g. the study protocol) required to understand and report research findings.
7. The authors should take responsibility for the way in which research findings are presented and published, be fully involved at all stages of publication and presentation development, and be willing to take public responsibility for all aspects of the work.
8. Author lists and contributorship statements should accurately reflect all substantial intellectual contributions to the research, data analyses, and publication or presentation development. Relevant contributions from persons who did not qualify as authors should also be disclosed.
9. The role of the sponsor in the design, execution, analysis, reporting, and

177

funding (if applicable) of the research should be fully disclosed in all publications and presentations of the findings. Any involvement by persons or organizations with an interest (financial or nonfinancial) in the findings should also be disclosed.

10. All authors and contributors should disclose any relationships or potential competing interests relating to the research and its publication or presentation.

Battisti W, Wager E, Baltzer L *et al.* (2015) Good Publication Practice for communicating company-sponsored medical research: GPP3. *Ann Intern Med.* **163**: 461–4.

Index

Entries in **bold** denote tables.